Professionalism in Medicine

Critical Perspectives

Delese Wear
Julie M. Aultman
Editors

Professionalism in Medicine

Critical Perspectives

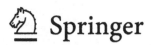 Springer

Editors:
Delese Wear, Julie M. Aultman
Northeastern Ohio Universities College of Medicine, U.S.A.

Library of Congress Cataloging-in-Publication Data

A C.I.P. Catalogue record for this book is available
from the Library of Congress.

ISBN 978-1-4419-4101-5   e-ISBN 10: 0-387-32727-4

                                          eISBN 13: 978-0-387-32727-3

Printed in the United States of America.

9 8 7 6 5 4 3 2 1

springer.com

CONTENTS

PART THREE

Assessing Professionalism

INTRODUCTION

Professionalism in Medicine: Critical Perspectives casts a careful, and at times wary, eye on a dominant force in contemporary academic medicine that appears to have been accepted as an absolute good. Calls for developing, increasing, or maintaining professionalism—not to mention the current obsession with evaluating or assessing it—appear with regularity in medical journals and conference programs of all stripes. The resultant literature has defined, organized, contained, and made seemingly immutable a group of attitudes and behaviors subsumed under the label "professional" or "professionalism" (Wear & Kuczewski, 2004). Moreover, the fixation with assessment has become a new steering mechanism that is reductionistic when it shapes the total range of possible and thinkable dimensions of professionalism. The richness, complexity, and contradictions of professionalism in medicine are being flattened into categorical attitudes or behaviors that evaluators (whose professionalism is rarely assessed) can check. As Mark Kuczewski, one of the contributors to this volume, observes, "Valuing and evaluating professionalism seem to have become equated."

This preoccupation with assessment is not indigenous to medical education. It is arising and taking hold of many institutions as new principles—indeed, mandates—of scrutiny and examination become acceptable, if not desirable, cultural practices. In their incisive work on audit cultures in higher education, Shore and Wright (2000) argue that coercive practices of accountability sometimes sound eerily like moves toward "exhibiting" professionalism whereby "every individual is made acutely aware that [his] conduct and performance is under constant scrutiny" (p. 77). This, it seems, is the direction of the professionalism movement in academic medicine, one that focuses on attitudes and behaviors that can be taught or sometimes modeled and thus evaluated like any other type of expertise or "competence." Moreover, audit cultures are interested in systems that track and indicate evidence of professional development (e.g., professional portfolios), so that medical students can become "auditable." Such constant surveillance for evidence or lack of professionalism becomes, according to Foucault (1977), a means to ensure that students constantly scrutinize themselves for confirmation that they have adopted the norms of conduct desired by the institutions educating them. The "more difficult (and politically charged) professionalism project of re-negotiating the social contract between physicians, communities, and other occupational groups"—that is, viewing professionalism as going to the heart of medical institutions, the profession itself, rather than unloading it on the individual student's or resident's shoulders—is rarely part of the conversation circulating in medical schools, associations, and other accrediting bodies (Shirley & Padgett in this volume).

In our quest for educating virtuous, sensitive, and skilled physicians it seems we have acceded, again, to the sirens of "economy over ecology, counting over accountability, objectivity over subjectivity, answers over questions, rigor over vitality, conclusions over curiosity, reduction over production, prose over poetry, reason over emotion, fragmentation over wholeness" (Leggo, 2005). Moreover, we have ceased careful consideration of what we're doing once "on board" the professionalism train. The authors here seek to slow down (if not stop) the train, asking difficult questions of us all. Their questioning is richly diverse and sometimes at odds with each other. They all agree that the issues underlying the recent calls for professionalism within medicine deserve focused attention, but that may be one of the few points of convergence. Each unravels, some more than others, the tidy package of professionalism that is often presented in the academic medicine literature.

In a much-needed, circumspect pause, this collection is the work of scholars who critically examine the current professionalism "movement" from various angles. We divide their essays into three major organizers: professionalism as a conceptual issue, a curricular issue, and a competency/assessment issue. However, we are quick to point out that these categories have permeable borders: Each essay is theoretically situated, each has curricular implications (even if not stated outright), and each has something to suggest about the role of assessment. Still, each essay seems to emerge from a particular critical location regarding one of these aspects of professionalism.

The first section, *professionalism as a conceptual issue*, provides readers with a convincing argument that conceptions of professionalism arise from multiple, diverse, and sometimes conflicting theoretical orientations. In the first chapter, "The Complexities of Medical Professionalism," Brian Castellani and Fred Hafferty offer a radical rethinking of professionalism by suggesting that there is not one but seven clusters of professionalism circulating in medicine. These clusters, which arise from different ways of organizing medical work, include nostalgic, unreflective, academic, entrepreneurial, empirical, lifestyle, and activist professionalism, and provide medical educators with a paradigm-shattering way to think about what they expect of, encourage, and assess students in terms of professional "growth." In their chapter, "An Analysis of the Discourse of Professionalism," Jamie Shirley and Stephen Padgett examine the professionalism movement through its language, using a post-structural analysis that recognizes language as a social practice. "Through language," they write, "communities reproduce their structures, discipline their members, and enact social practices." Their position, one that radically departs from current convention, is that professionalism efforts miss the boat because they "locate the solutions to systematic problems of medical education and practice in the virtues of individual physicians." The third chapter in this section represents a traditional approach to professionalism in academic medicine. David Doukas's "Professionalism: Curriculum Goals and Meeting Their Challenges" begins with the assumption that the recent mandates for professionalism by the LCME and ACGME represent the best standards to which professionalism efforts should aspire. As a means to put these high standards into action, he presents a model code of professionalism for medical students, residents, and their teachers that will be formally and openly expressed at various junctures in the medical education process. Hopefully, readers will be struck with the wide theoretical divergence of these three perspectives on professionalism.

Professionalism as a curricular issue is the largest section of the book. Here authors elaborate on the content, pedagogy, and placement of professionalism in the medical curriculum, and here also are points of agreement and major divergence. Daniel George, Iahn Gonsenhauser and Peter Whitehouse posit in "The Nature of Story and the Story of Nature" that professionalism efforts have largely been "more of a humanizing veneer of platitudes and abstract definitions than an operational ethos in students' lives." Proposing that professional development must conjoin medical and public health, they recommend course work based on a narrative approach where students take a central role in their own exploration of scientific and ethical values. Delese Wear focuses more narrowly on one element of professionalism—respect—and develops a curriculum based on a "pedagogy of discomfort" in her chapter, "Respect for Patients: A Case Study of the Formal and Hidden Curriculum." In place of professionalism, Jack Coulehan suggests a more comprehensive approach, a "rebirth of medical morality for the 21st century." In its current iteration, professionalism "avoids grappling with deep issues of value and character formation and fails to internalize the narrative tradition of medicine." At the end his chapter, "You Say Self-Interest, I Say Altruism," he demonstrates how fictional narratives can contribute to the character formation of medical students.

While each arises from different perspectives, all three of the aforementioned chapters look to literature and other narrative forms. The next three chapters emphasize the need to step back and take a critical look at the language and curricular practices of professionalism. In her chapter "The Role of Ethics within Professionalism Inquiry," Julie Aultman argues that the language of professionalism is imprecise, if not inaccurate, when conflated with medical ethics. She notes that even among medical educators these areas of inquiry and application are poorly understood and are ostensibly taught under the misguided assumption that the *theoretical* underpinnings of professional and ethical values and concepts are of no importance in medical education. Aultman identifies significant distinctions in the approaches and goals between professionalism inquiry and medical ethics, providing clear definitions and methodologies for each, along with practice-based boundaries between the two. Similar to the theoretical position taken by Jamie Shirley and Steve Padgett in the first section of this book, Brad Lewis strongly argues in his chapter, "Medical Professionals and the Discourse of Professionalism," that the discourse of professionalism should be reworked to include a meaningful distinction between "the institution of medicine as a *social* phenomenon and the professionalism movement as largely focused on *individual* physicians." Curricular implications here focus on "teaching the conflicts" in professionalism whereby educators bring to the forefront the incommensurabilities embedded in the profession by exposing students to critical scholarship that identifies the deep problems and contradictions in contemporary medical systems. Finally, Thomas Inui and colleagues describe a dramatic, systemic, environmental change that "attempts to change the culture of a large medical school and, therefore, align the formal and the informal curricula." Their chapter, "Educating for Professionalism at Indiana University School of Medicine," delineates how professionalism education takes place in a competency-directed curriculum, and like other competencies, "is considered to be an explicit objective of every required experience a student has at IUSM."

Four chapters complete the last section of the book, which focuses on *professionalism as a competency/assessment issue.* In "The Problem with Evaluating Professionalism," Mark Kuczewski elaborates on just that: "The desire for objective assessment is determining how medical education construes professionalism." To that end, the most seemingly objective assessments are those more likely to document unacceptable behaviors rather than to encourage positive ones. And rather than focus all attention on the former, he suggests ways to demonstrate how medical educators value professionalism in the medical school and clinical environments. Cynthia Brincat, a philosopher turned physician, provides a critically reflective first-person account of the professionalism efforts she has experienced and observed as a student and resident. In her chapter, "How Medical Training Mangles Professionalism," Brincat develops the idea that the "professionalism crisis in medicine is, in many ways, manufactured." Moreover, she argues, this "disease" model of professionalism actually divorces it from compassion, "its deepest root and spring." Audiey Kao and Jennifer Reenan offer another perspective in their chapter, "*Wit* is Not Enough." They argue that professionalism education is failing because there is low demand for it and the quality of its efforts are of questionable value. Their solution is not to offer more humanities courses but to "redefine professionalism in a manner that reaffirms the interdependent nature of the art and science of medicine," particularly in curricular, instructional, and assessment efforts. They offer eight "design principles" for professionalism education, most of which rest on a belief that there are indeed "professionalism competencies." Finally, Laura Fochtmann offers a comprehensive assessment of efforts to "measure" professionalism and the implications of those measurements for students, faculty and patients. Her chapter, "Professionalism and the Heisenberg Uncertainty Principle," provides a thoughtful look at the "pitfalls in evaluation of professionalism" and calls for medical educators to break their "addiction to measurement," which would allow us to focus time and efforts on professionalism in a more positive, global sense. The collection ends with the thoughtful observations and recommendations of David Leach, Executive Director of the Accreditation Council for Graduate Medical Education.

Our intent in this introduction is to prepare readers to expect writing that is marked by critical theorizing, that asks unexpected questions, and that goes against the grain. As Mark Kuczewski notes in his chapter, "We should never hesitate to say things that fly in the face of the received wisdom." These authors do not hesitate, and it is our hope that their words inspire us all to think about what we are doing. Maxine Greene, philosopher and educator, has spent a lifetime encouraging others to resist the notion of a finished, predetermined, objective reality. We take up her preoccupation here, providing a space "for the articulation of multiple perspectives in multiple idioms, out of which something common can be brought into being" (Greene, 1988, p. xi).

REFERENCES

Greene, M. (1988). *The dialectic of freedom.* New York: Teachers College Press.
Leggo, C. (2005). Attending to winter: A poetics of research. Paper presented at the American Educational Research Association, Montreal, CA.
Shore, C., & Wright, S. (2000). Coercive accountability: The rise of audit culture in higher education. In M. Strathern (Ed.), *Audit cultures: Anthropological studies in accountability, ethics and the academy* (pp. 75-89). London: Routledge.

Part One

CONCEPTUALIZING PROFESSIONALISM

Chapter 1

THE COMPLEXITIES OF MEDICAL PROFESSIONALISM
A Preliminary Investigation

Brian Castellani
Kent State University

Frederic W. Hafferty
University of Minnesota-Duluth, School of Medicine

INTRODUCTION

Efforts within organized medicine over the last twenty years to re-establish an ethic of professionalism have obscured the fact that currently there are several competing clusters or types of medical professionalism, each of which represents a unique approach to medical work. Stated differently, the "professionalism" that has emerged within the academic medical journals, conferences, debates, and discussions over the past twenty years is a highly selective and privileged narrative, developed and delivered by one, possibly two, particular strata within the organizational structure of medicine. We call this strata the ruling class of medicine, and we refer to its medical professionalism as *nostalgic*. The other clusters of medical professionalism that we empirically "discovered" include *entrepreneurial*, *empirical*, *lifestyle*, *unreflective*, *academic*, and *activist* professionalism.

The development of this seven-cluster system of medical professionalism was by no means an accident. Instead, it was the direct result of our involvement in the new science of complexity (e.g., Axelrod, 1997; Bak, 1999; Capra, 1996; Cilliers, 1998; Holland, 1998). Specifically, we are in the process of developing our own theoretical and methodological framework, which we applied to the current study.

The purpose of this chapter is to introduce readers to a more "complex" medical professionalism. To do so, we begin with a quick overview of the theory and method we developed, along with the historical archive we used to conduct our empirical analyses. Next, we review the five important ways the theory and method helped us to recognize, discover, analyze and assemble medical professionalism as a complex social system, including a thick description of the seven clusters we discovered. We conclude by putting the complex social system of medical professionalism together, reflecting on the insights our results have for the future teaching and evaluation of professionalism.

IS PROFESSIONALISM REALLY THAT COMPLEX?

Over the last twenty years, an entirely new way of doing science has emerged, which many leading scholars are heralding as a critical scientific paradigm of the 21st century (e.g., Capra, 1996, 2002; Kauffman, 2000). The name of this new paradigm is *complexity science* (e.g., Bar-Yam, 1997; Byrne, 1998; Waldrop, 1992). Complexity science has become part of the intellectual imagination through a series of mainstream academic works that have popularized this new science's core topics, including complex adaptive systems (e.g., Holland, 1995), chaos theory (Gleick, 1987), fractal geometry (Mandelbrot, 1983), computer-based modeling (Casti, 1999; Holland 1998), self-organizing systems (Kauffman, 2000), artificial life (Ward, 1999), and complex networks (Barabási, 2002; Watts, 1999).

In medicine, research into complexity science's core topics has led to a number of important advances. In epidemiology, for example, this research has provided a very sophisticated way of mapping and studying how diseases are transmitted globally and locally through the various social networks in which people live and work (e.g., Barabási, 2002); in biomedical research it has led to new computational techniques for modeling the complexities of biological systems (e.g., Kauffman, 2000; Ward, 1999); in family medicine it has helped to better understand the dynamics of group medical practice (e.g., Aita, McIlvain, Susman, & Crabtree, 2003; Miller, Reuben, McDaniel, Crabtree, & Stange, 2001); in health care management it has led to a more sophisticated understanding of the complexities of professional organizations and their management (e.g., Anderson & McDaniel, 2000; McDaniel, Jordan, & Fleeman, 2003); and in qualitative health research it has led to the development of a whole new set of techniques (e.g., Agar, 2003; Anderson, Crabtree, Steele, & McDaniel, 2005; Castellani, Castellani & Spray, 2003; Castellani & Castellani, 2003).

Social Complexity Theory and Assemblage

The theory and method we used for this study are called, respectively, *social complexity theory* and *assemblage*. Their conjoint purpose is to help researchers recognize, discover, analyze and assemble various social phenomena as complex social systems. Social complexity theory does this by providing researchers a useful set of concepts that explain how complex social systems work. Assemblage does this by showing researchers how to discover and analyze a complex social system by building it from the ground up.

In terms of the current study, social complexity theory and assemblage helped us in five important ways: 1) to realize and discover medical professionalism as a complex system; 2) to develop a historical database for its study; 3) to determine the field of relations in which it has been situated for the last thirty years; 4) to assemble its internal organization into ten key aspects of medical work; and 5) to discover and develop our seven-cluster network of professionalism.

MAKING PROFESSIONALISM COMPLEX

The first way social complexity theory and assemblage helped was enabling us to realize and discover medical professionalism as a complex system. Our decision to pursue the current study was the result of a series of conversations we had about medical professionalism and complexity science. During these conversations we repeatedly asked ourselves a basic question: "Is the current discourse on professionalism truly singular and totalizing, or is it 'privileged,' meaning that there are other ways of practicing medical professionalism but they are hidden or overshadowed by the current dominant discourse?"

During our conversations two issues in particular suggested the latter: the increasing relevance that lifestyle and personal morality seem to play in the professional behavior of medical students and medical residents (e.g., Rippe, 1999; Wear & Castellani, 2002), and the extent to which the professionalism of practicing physicians seems to be infused with an "entrepreneurial" spirit (e.g. Hafferty, 2005). It appeared to us that both of these factors were not just diminishing the current discourse on professionalism, but seemed to be the basis for entirely new ways of practicing professionalism. Inspired by these initial insights, we began to build our database.

ARCHIVING THE DISCOURSE ON PROFESSIONALISM

The primary data for our study was the discourse on medical professionalism, which included the professional dominance, deprofessionalization and medical professionalism literature, as well as any published empirical studies on the professional behavior of medical students, medical residents and physicians. It also included letters to the editors, reviews and reports published and/or distributed by such leading organizations as the American Board of Internal Medicine (ABIM), the Association of American Medical Colleges (AAMC), the Accreditation Council on Graduate Medical Education (ACGME), the National Board of Medical Examiners (NBME), and the Liaison Committee on Medical Education's (LCME). Additional materials came from articles, commentaries, responses and related material dealing with medical professionalism that were found in various medical sociology journals and more popular U.S. publications such as *The New Yorker*, *The Wall Street Journal*, and *The New York Times*. Following Foucault's methodological guidelines for conducting an investigation into the history of ideas (1980), we treated all the discourses on medical professionalism as historical data for sociological study.

BEYOND THE RISE AND FALL OF MEDICINE

With our basic question and archive in hand, the theory and method helped us determine the set of external forces that have pushed organized medicine into a state of increasing professional complexity. In complexity science a distinction is commonly made between the external and internal state of a complex social system (e.g., Capra, 1996; Klir, 2001; Luhmann, 1995; Maturana & Varela, 1992). The external state can be thought of as the larger field of relations within which a complex social system is situated. This distinction is important because what researchers have consistently found is that the internal dynamics of a complex social system are primarily dependent upon the external forces impacting the system as a whole (Capra, 1996). In other words, changes taking place within a complex social system often are due to changes taking place in the external environment (e.g., Geyer & Zouwen, 2001; Luhmann, 1995). In the case of medical professionalism, we concluded that the seven clusters of medical professionalism we discovered emerged in direct response to the historical forces of decentralization in which organized medicine has been situated for the last thirty years. An abridged version of this story is as follows.

Every graduate student specializing in medical sociology is introduced at some level to the following storyline of 20th century American medicine, as told by sociology. This sociological story begins early in the 20th century with Carr-Saunders and Wilson's *The Professions* (1933/1964). This phase is known as the reform and initial rise of organized medicine, and is characterized by a period of profound and rapid development during which medicine not only grew in scientific and technical competence, but also in status and legitimacy (e.g., Starr, 1982). The second phase, which begins around the 1940s and continues onward through the 1960s, is known as medicine's phase of professional dominance. As analytically dissected in Eliot's Freidson's twin classics, *Professional Dominance* (1970) and *Profession of Medicine* (1970), organized medicine rose to the top of health care system and the professional class pyramid between the 1940s and the 1960s by controlling the production of medical knowledge, exercising authority over the division of medical labor, supervising and regulating the provision of health services, and maintaining control over the organization of medicine and the health care system. Additionally, medicine gained economic, political and cultural power by continuing to convince the economic and governmental elites, as well as the general population, that what it did as a profession was both valuable and necessary and required little to no outside regulation.

The 1960s, however, brought a whole new set of challenges that organized medicine, despite all of its efforts, was unable to effectively counter. These challenges included the skyrocketing costs of health care; the transformation of medicine from a cottage industry to a corporate "player" on Wall Street; the emergence of Medicare, Medicaid, and managed health care; the corporatization of medicine, which turned medical knowledge and treatment into a commodity; the patient-consumerism movement; the rise and competition of other health care professions (e.g., nursing, physician-assistants, etc); advances in medical and biomedical technology; cultural and academic challenges to the professional legitimacy of medicine; and the computer and information revolution, which increased the surveillance of physicians by various bureaucratic formations, including the federal government, evidence-based medicine, patient safety, physician report cards, health insurance panels, review boards, accrediting agencies, hospital administrations, and patient and intellectual watch-groups.

Within the medical sociology literature, this complex set of factors represent the third phase of medicine's history (e.g., Hafferty & McKinlay, 1993; Hafferty & Light, 1995), which medical sociologists describe as one of deprofessionalization (Haug, 1988), proletarianization (McKinlay & Arches, 1985) and corporatization (e.g., McKinlay & Stoeckle 1980). In this essay, we group all of these challenges under the single heading, *forces of decentralization.*

Establishing the forces of decentralization as our larger field of relations, we arrived at the following (albeit tentative) conclusion. For the last thirty years organized medicine has been situated within a larger field of relations that has consistently and rather successfully challenged its longstanding position of professional dominance. In response to these forces of decentralization, physicians began to practice other types of professionalism, which lead to the development and emergence of several competing clusters of medical professionalism. This is not to say that some of these clusters did not exist prior to this phase. In fact, it is entirely reasonable that even during the first half of the 20th century, when the narrative of "nostalgic professionalism" was dominant, that there might have been several other clusters of professionalism. What changed in the third phase, however, was that the forces of decentralization massively decreased the ruling class's position of power, allowing for the emergence and growth of several already existing and newly forming clusters, specifically entrepreneurial, empirical, and lifestyle professionalism.

The problem, as we see it, is that because the ruling class of medicine has so desperately spent the last thirty years fighting the forces of decentralization, it has not realized that its campaign to re-establish professionalism has not only been challenged by the larger systems of which it is a part, it has not even been embraced by many of its own members, the rank-and-file of medicine. In fact, many physicians, such as those practicing an entrepreneurial, empirical, lifestyle or activist professionalism, *reject* the traditional tenets of nostalgic professionalism. These alternative forms of professionalism have been supported in their resistance by the larger social forces of which they are a part, which include the corporatization of medicine, the newly emerging culture of the professional class and generation X, the feminization of medicine, the continued problems of health care costs and third-party insurance, and the economically troubled state of the federal government. In short, medical professionalism is not what it used to be; it is, in fact, a whole new and very complex social system.

PROFESSIONALISM AS MEDICAL WORK

With the historical forces of decentralization established as our larger field of relations, the next thing social complexity theory and assemblage helped us do was arrange the internal organization of medical professionalism. In

Table 1. The Seven Competing Clusters of Medical Professionalism

	Nostalgic	Entrepreneurial	Academic	Lifestyle	Empirical	Unreflective	Activist
Most Important	Autonomy Altruism Interpersonal Competence Personal Morality Professional Dominance Technical Competence	Commercialism Autonomy Technical Competence Professional Dominance	Altruism Interpersonal Competence Technical Competence Lifestyle	Autonomy Lifestyle Personal Morality	Autonomy Technical Competence Commercialism Professional Dominance Altruism	Autonomy Interpersonal Competence Personal Morality Altruism	Social Justice Social Contract Altruism Personal Morality
Moderately Important	Social Contract Social Justice	Lifestyle Personal Morality	Personal Morality Professional Dominance Social Contract Autonomy	Commercialism Interpersonal Competence Technical Competence	Social Contract Personal Morality	Technical Competence Lifestyle Professional Dominance	Interpersonal Competence Technical Competence Autonomy
Least Important	Lifestyle Commercialism	Lifestyle Altruism Social Justice Social Contract	Social Justice Commercialism	Altruism Social Contract Social Justice Professional Dominance	Social Justice Interpersonal Competence Lifestyle	Commercialism Social Justice Social Contract	Lifestyle Commercialism Professional Dominance

terms of a complex system's internal state, it is common practice in complexity to make a distinction between organization and dynamics (e.g., Capra, 1996; Luhmann, 1995; Maturana & Varela, 1992). Organization refers to the various parts, elements or components that contribute to a complex social system's internal structure. We call this internal organization or structure the *web of subsystems*, which emphasizes Luhmann's important point that these components are systems in and of themselves (1995). At this point, a caveat is necessary. While the internal organization of a complex social system is "real," it also involves an intellectual entity. As in traditional scientific research, it is the complexity scientist's job to decide what subsystems are relevant and why. This is done through empirical inquiry of one type or another—historical, statistical, qualitative, computational. Whatever the technique used, the goal is to create a list of subsystems that, when put together, allow the researcher to understand adequately the organization of the complex social system of study.

We decided to explain the organization of medical professionalism in terms of what we considered to be ten key aspects of medical work. Our rationale for doing so is based on our training as medical sociologists. Unlike many scholars in academic medicine who conceptualize professionalism as a set of values or "value orientations," we see it as a way of organizing work, such that an occupation can claim the status of profession (Freidson, 2001). Some of these ways of organizing work amount to specific value orientations (as in the case of altruism) or beliefs (as in the case of social justice), while others represent specific skills (such as technical or interpersonal competence) or ways of controlling the position of an occupation within the larger bureaucratic structure of which it is a part (as in the case of autonomy and professional dominance).

As shown in Table 1 (see page 20), the ten key aspects of medical work that we arrived at, and our basic working definitions of them, are as follows. *Autonomy* is defined as discretionary decision-making; i.e., you do your work the way you think it should be done (e.g., Hsia, 2001; Schneider, 1998). *Commercialism* is the application of business principles to medical practice and the turning of medical knowledge into a commodity (e.g., Bodenheimer, 1999; Lindorf, 1992). *Social justice* is the idea of medicine as fairness (e.g., Daniels, Light, & Caplan, 1996). *Social contract* is the covenant between medicine and society with reciprocal rights and obligations (e.g., Caelleigh, 2001; Coulehan, Williams, Van McCrary, & Belling, 2003). *Altruism* is placing the welfare of patients ahead of one's own (e.g., McGaghie, Mytko, Brown, & Cameron, 2002; Schiedermayer & McCarthy, 1995). *Professional dominance* describes an organizational arrangement where medicine is in a position of control over the organization, delivery and payment of health care (e.g., Freidson, 1970a, 1970b; Hafferty & McKinlay, 1993). *Technical competence* and *interpersonal competence* refer to the possession of the appropriate skills related to diagnosing, treating and communicating well with patients and others. *Lifestyle ethic* is the devaluation of work in relationship to personal and family life (e.g., Rippe, 1999; Schwartz, Jarecky, Strodel, Haley, Young, & Griffen, 1989). *Personal morality* is one's own personal (as opposed to professional) belief system (e.g., Fox, Arnold, & Brody, 1995).

THE COMPETING CLUSTERS OF PROFESSIONALISM

The fifth way social complexity theory and assemblage helped us was in conceptualizing the *internal dynamics* of medical professionalism. Dynamics refers to the processes by which the agents in a complex social system use the web of subsystems to create, organize, and change the system in response to the demands of the external environment. Complexity scientists use a variety of terms, some new and some old, to describe these agent-based processes, including emergence, evolution, adaptation, feedback, autopoiesis, perturbation, self-organization, and operating far from equilibrium (Capra, 1996, 2002; Cilliers, 1998; Holland, 1998; Geyer and Zouwen, 2001).

In terms of the current study, this terminology helped us understand three important things about the internal dynamics of medical professionalism. First, as shown in Table 1, it helped us understand the different ways that American physicians have organized the ten subsystems of medical work in response to the historical forces of decentralization. For each cluster we rank ordered the ten subsystems of medical work in terms of their relative importance to the physicians within the cluster, with the most important at the top and the least important at the bottom. Because our identification and ordering of the clusters are not based on any particular subsystem, we decided to group the ten subsystems for each cluster into three basic sets: most important, moderately important and least important.

Second, the terminology on dynamics helped us understand the clusters of medical professionalism created by these different ways of organizing medical work. As shown in Table 1, our preliminary analysis revealed seven competing clusters of professionalism—nostalgic, unreflective, academic, entrepreneurial, empirical, lifestyle, and activist—each of which represents a unique way of combining and practicing what we identified as the ten ideals of medical work.

Third, the terminology of dynamics helped us understand the entirely new system of medical professionalism that has emerged over the past ten to fifteen years as a function of the interactions between these competing clusters of professionalism. The purpose of the final section of our chapter addresses this third issue as we focus on describing the seven clusters.

Nostalgic Professionalism and the Ruling Class

The ruling class of medicine is made up of those individuals, groups and organizations that hold an elite status within organized medicine, including the leaders of academic medicine and medical education, the editors of many of the first-tier medical journals such as *Academic Medicine, The New England Journal of Medicine,* and the *Annals of Internal Medicine,* along with various organizations and groups such as the American Board of Internal Medicine (ABIM) and the Association of American Medical Colleges (AAMC), the Accreditation Council on Graduate Medical Education (ACGME), the American Medical Association (AMA), and the Liaison Committee on Medical Education's (LCME). We call this group the ruling class because their positions of privilege and authority have afforded them to have a profound influence on the academic discourse of medical professionalism over the past thirty years, so much so that their nostalgic professionalism has become *the* discourse of medical professionalism, one that is "used by administrators, clinical faculty, residency programs, and professional organizations with the expectation of shared meanings and goals" (Wear & Kuczewski, 2004, p. 1).

We call the ruling class's professionalism nostalgic because their campaign—which Wear and Kuczewski call a social movement (2004)—does not advocate a new professionalism, one that reflects the profound external changes and challenges facing organized medicine. Instead, it advocates (attempts to re-establish) a "professionalism of old" for which they long—a professionalism that is grounded in autonomy and dominance and that houses an immense disdain for commercialism. It is within this narrative that commercialism is most unilaterally cast as the antithesis and enemy of "medical professionalism." Their solution is to re-establish professional dominance over it. In this way, nostalgic professionalism is conventional, mainstream medical professionalism, as it has been idealized by organized medicine and the social sciences for the past hundred years (e.g., Starr, 1982).

Academic Professionalism

Closely aligned with the medicine's ruling class are those physicians practicing academic professionalism (e.g., Starr, 1982). Like the majority of the ruling class, these physicians also work in academic medical centers, medical schools, and related medical organizations. And like the ruling class, they have been involved in the nostalgic professionalism movement. However, the similarity ends here.

The main difference is that, unlike the ruling elite, academics are the rank-and-file of academic medicine. These are the thousands of physician faculty who teach and care for patients within the medical school-residency system, which more recently includes the responsibilities of evaluating their students according to the new professionalism competencies mandated by the ACGME. Yet, for all their work with professionalism, it is not really their battle. Instead, professionalism is one more thing they have to juggle in their daily regiment of teaching and clinical practice. It is for this reason that, while they rank altruism high and commercialism low, they do not place much stock in issues of autonomy or professional dominance. For them, while the forces of decentralization (particularly commercialization) are an issue, the professionalism campaign is strictly an academic affair and is therefore low on their list of things about which to worry (e.g., Coulehan & Williams, 2003).

Entrepreneurial Professionalism

In almost direct opposition to nostalgic professionalism stands entrepreneurial professionalism. Interestingly enough, while this cluster has grown in significance over the past twenty years, it is not new. As any historian of medicine knows, there has always been an entrepreneurial element to medical work and there have always been physicians who have practiced medicine as a business (e.g., Brown, 1979; Lewis, 1925/1998; Starr, 1982). In fact, this entrepreneurial spirit was the commercialism that organized medicine sought to get rid of—with considerable success—during the late 1800s and early 1900s. What changed in the 1980s was Wall Street's discovery of clinical medicine as a profit center, which re-invigorated an ethic of commercialism in the examination and operating rooms of clinical medicine, legitimating the desire of a significant number of physicians to ground their professionalism in the ethics of business. And so was born entrepreneurial professionalism (e.g., Hafferty, 2004, 2005).

Entrepreneurial professionalism is comprised of physicians from just about every area of medicine, ranging from physicians who started their own specialty surgery or imaging centers to those practicing boutique and retainer medicine, to those performing vanity plastic surgery or selling Amway products in their offices (e.g., Hafferty, 2005). Despite these differences, the theme of this cluster is consistent. In the past thirty years, the costs of health care have skyrocketed, patients are not as safe as they should be, too many patients have no or poor health care insurance, and too many physicians fail to practice according to the evidence. By grounding the organization, delivery, and payment of health care in the principles of business, entrepreneurial professionalism—at least as an ideal type—can fix these problems, guarantee a better product to a larger number of patient-consumers, and do so at a cheaper price. This, they believe, will lead to a better health care system for everyone.

Lifestyle Professionalism

Riding on the back of entrepreneurial professionalism is the newest and youngest of the seven competing clusters: lifestyle professionalism (e.g., Rippe, 1999). Lifestyle professionalism is the culmination of some of the most important economic, cultural and political changes of the last forty years. In addition to the forces of decentralization, it includes the civil rights movement, the counterculture movement of the 1960s and 1970s, the rise of professional class culture, the feminization of medicine, the environmental movement, and the emergence of the postmodern, global society in which we now live. Its most immediate force, however, is entrepreneurial professionalism because, without the proliferation of new practice opportunities, including the possibility of working in a shared practice, a salaried part-time position, or as a *locum tenems*, lifestyle physicians would not be able to practice the alternative forms of work in which they are interested.

The physicians practicing lifestyle professionalism range from part-time female physician-mothers (e.g., Wear & Castellani, 2001) to physicians interested in working with fewer patients, that is, those who simply do not want to work that hard. The majority of physicians in this cluster represent the latter. Despite these differences in outlook and motivation, the general age and theme of lifestyle professionals are the same. These are younger physicians (usually under 40) who believe that nostalgic professionalism over-emphasizes work at the exclusion of other values and social institutions—such as personal and family life, friends, marriage, physical and mental health, hobbies and even fun. They believe that the current workaholic attitude of traditional medicine is bad for the health and well-being of physicians and their patients. As such, lifestyle professionalism is all about "balance." Even when it comes to altruism, for example, lifestyle professionals believe there should be a balance between one's self and the needs of one's patients. For some, this means that one must take care of oneself *before* one can adequately care for others. In either case, lifestyle professionals believe that their approach to professionalism leads to a win-win situation for everyone (e.g., Rippe, 1999; Schwartz, Jarecky, Strodel, Haley, Young, & Griffen, 1989; Wear & Castellani, 2002).

Empirical Professionalism

Empirical professionalism is the alter ego of academic professionalism. Like its brethren, empirical professionalism houses/captures those academic physicians whose function is as physician/academic-researchers, as opposed to physician/academic clinicians. Similar to their counterparts, academic researchers have been professionalism players since the mid to late 1800s. Initially, they were the "gentleman-physicians" who dabbled in their home laboratories (e.g., Lewis, 1925/1998). Following World War II, and with the advent of the National Institutes of Health (NIH), these physicians became an important part of the academic medical center. Once again, it was not until the 1980s, when Wall Street began to embrace biomedical research on a broad scale that empirical professionalism took on a shape of its own (see Starr, 1982).

Unlike the other clusters, empirical professionalism is a smaller and more homogeneous group of physician-researchers who see themselves (and often are treated) as occupying the top of the academic medicine pyramid. They are the ones who are responsible for creating new medical knowledge and tools. Because of their belief in the ultimate benefit of their ideas, autonomy and technical competence are ranked high, but then so is commercialism and their assumed "right" to benefit from their discoveries. Because academic medical centers are so dependent upon the prestige and indirect costs they generate through grants, and because so much of this research depends upon multi-million dollar research funding, empirical professionals have a pragmatic understanding of the importance of generating money. And so they have emerged as a major contender in the field of medical professionalism.

Unreflective Professionalism

The sixth major cluster is unreflective professionalism. The physicians who occupy this cluster are the older rank-and-file community/street physicians. They are not researchers, activists, or entrepreneurs. Nor do not work in academic medicine, publish articles or place high priority on issues of lifestyle. They are however, the traditional backbone of the health care delivery system in the United States. They keep their nose close to the clinical practice grindstone, knowing (and sometimes, even caring) little about the "big issues" coursing through medicine. These are the physicians who get up every day, go to their offices, and treat patients. Their lack of involvement in the whole dynamic of re-establishing or resisting the nostalgic professionalism of the ruling class is why we refer to them as "unreflective." In fact, many of them are not even aware that any sort of "professionalism" movement is taking place. It is also for this reason that they have almost no voice in the academic medicine literature.

This does not mean, however, that the forces of decentralization do not seriously challenge them. As the primary providers of care, they live the daily struggles of work in a complex health care system and, as such, they are very concerned about issues of commercialism, autonomy, altruism and competence. Their lack of input to the "formal" professionalism discourse, however, condemns them to a certain marginal status within the professionalism campaign. They are not concerned about debating definitions, creating measurement schemes, evaluating the professionalism of students, or of patenting the next big discovery in bio-technological medicine and thus the next hot start-up company. Instead, they are primarily concerned with staying afloat with respect to practice economics, practice knowledge and skills, and practice value orientations. There is nothing "cutting edge" about them.

Activist Professionalism

Of the seven clusters presented here, the most consistent in size and stature over time (tracing all the way back to the early 1900s), is activist professionalism (Starr, 1982). Basically, this is a historically small and ideologically focused group. They also, with respect to the currents of traditional professionalism, are a rather marginalized group (e.g., Brown, 1979; Burrow, 1977). Because of their small group size and homogeneous value system, this cluster is composed both of rank-and-file physician activists, along with those like Paul Farmer (2003), Howard Waitzkin (1991) and David Hilfiker (2002) who have found a media outlet (academic or popular) for their views. Physician activists range from those who work in public health and community medicine to those who provide medical care for underrepresented and underserved populations to those who campaign for national health care (e.g., Physicians for a National Health Program).

The dominant concern of this cluster is social justice. They take their Hippocratic Oath very seriously, believing that medicine is not a business, a research institute, an elite occupation, a lifestyle, or a way to rise in income, status or power. Instead, they believe in *living* their commitment to their patients and to society to provide the care that is needed. It is for these reasons that they place high priority on social justice, social contract and altruism, and rank low the issues of commercialism, lifestyle and professional dominance. There is, however, a critical irony here. These are the physicians who best exemplify, in terms of their daily work, the ideas and ideals of self-less professionalism. These are the altruists. At the same time, activist physicians are generally seen by their peers as professionally deviant. It is for this reason that we refer to them as activists: it makes it clear that their *level* of commitment to the health and well-being of patients is politically, economically, culturally, and, most important, organizationally outside the boundaries of what is considered professionally mainstream.

ASSEMBLING THE SYSTEM

Now that we have a basic understanding of how we went about conceptualizing medical professionalism as a complex social system, it is time to put everything together. We began this study with a critical question. We wanted to know if the ruling class's efforts within organized medicine over the last twenty years to re-establish an ethic of professionalism have obscured the possibility that physicians today practice more than one type of medical professionalism. To answer this question, we turned to the sociology of complexity (e.g., Geyer & Zouwen, 2001), specifically social complexity theory and the method of assemblage, which we are currently developing to help researchers study the complex dynamics of many social phenomena (Castellani & Hafferty, forthcoming).

Based on our empirical analyses, we concluded that for the last thirty years the professional dominance of U.S. has been consistently and rather successfully challenged by a series of decentralizing historical forces that go by the names of deprofessionalization, corporatization and proletarianization. More specifically, these forces have undermined the traditional professionalism of the ruling class of medicine, allowing for the rise in power and size of an alternative network of competing clusters. Still, for all of this change, it appears that the nostalgic professionalism of the ruling class currently maintains a position of dominance, particularly within academic medicine and medical education. But this may not be for long.

Remembering that these clusters of professionalism do not exist in isolation from one another, and that as a network they represent medical professionalism's response to the forces of decentralization, it is possible that entrepreneurial professionalism and lifestyle professionalism may be in a unique position to take over. The forces of decentralization, specifically commercialism, seem to be fueling their continual rise in size and power, particularly over the last ten years. This potential takeover may be further reinforced by the fact that the ruling class has done little to align itself with its more natural ally, activist professionalism. The ruling class also has failed to recognize the lifestyle professionalism of younger physicians, medical residents and students as a viable competing force. This is made further problematic by the potential of rank-and-file academic physicians to treat professionalism as a strictly academic affair and for the majority of older practicing physicians to remain on the sidelines in terms of recognizing or reflecting on what is happening.

Still, our results are preliminary. Further research needs to 1) examine our conceptualization of professionalism as medical work; 2) determine the empirical validity of the seven clusters we identified; 3) decide if any of these clusters overlap with each other or are comprised of a series of sub-clusters; and 4) examine the impact these competing clusters are having on each other and the system of medical professionalism as a whole.

Despite the need for additional research, we believe our basic tenet is foundational. While the exact number of competing clusters is open for debate, and while the ten subsystems may be modified or redefined, it is clear that more than one discourse of medical professionalism exists. It is on this basic point that we challenge the current literature on professionalism, particularly as it is applied to medical education.

TEACHING AND EVALUATING PROFESSIONALISM

The following are our recommendations for improving the future teaching and evaluation of medical students and residents. Because they are based on our preliminary results, future research should explore them further.

The Academic Medicine Literature

1. The current discourse on professionalism needs to be re-conceptualized to take into account the empirical fact that medical professionalism is a complex social system comprised of several competing clusters of professionalism.

2. As part of this re-conceptualization, scholars need to recognize that the current discourse on professionalism reflects the nostalgic professionalism of the ruling class.
3. Scholars writing from other perspectives, particularly those practicing an entrepreneurial, lifestyle and activist professionalism, need to be heard.
4. A voice also needs to be given to the struggles and viewpoints of the majority of older physicians practicing an unreflective professionalism.
5. Current measures for assessing professionalism need to retooled, if necessary, to assess the different types of professionalism physicians practice.
6. Scholars in the academic medicine literature need to integrate more fully their ideas with medical sociology in order to better conceptualize the impact the forces of decentralization are having on medical professionalism.

Medical Educators

1. Medical educators (i.e. administrators, clinical faculty, residency directors, preceptors, basic science faculty, etc.) need to become explicitly involved in the process of addressing the complexities of professionalism.
2. Seminars and other forms of evaluation need to be provided to medical educators to better understand a) their own views about the forces of decentralization, particularly commercialism, and b) the type of medical professionalism they practice.
3. Further research is needed to determine if and why the majority of clinical faculty treat the teaching and evaluation of professionalism as routine.
4. Further research is also needed to understand the different types of professionalism that clinical faculty (e.g., preceptors, adjuncts, etc.) may be unreflectively bringing to their interactions with students and residents.

Curriculum

1. The current curriculum needs to be assessed to determine the ways in which it "has defined, organized, contained, and made seemingly immutable a group of attitudes, values, and behaviors" at the expense of all other ways of practicing professionalism (Wear & Kuczewski, 2004, pp. 1-2).
2. Further research needs to explore how the forces of decentralization and the current competing clusters of medical professionalism are making

their way into medical education, particularly through the hidden curriculum.

Medical Students and Residents

1. Medical students and residents need to become explicitly involved in the process of addressing the complexities of professionalism.
2. Seminars, lectures, courses, and other forms of teaching and evaluation need to be provided to students and residents so they can understand a) their own views about the forces of decentralization, particularly commercialism, and b) the different types of professionalism they are interested in practicing.
3. To facilitate points one and two, medical educators need to help students identify—as early as the first year and then throughout their medical education—the different types of professionalism they are interested in practicing.
4. Medical educators also need to realize that students and residents are likely to view physicians who practice a nostalgic professionalism as patronizing, old-fashioned, outdated, and unhealthy.
5. Finally, medical educators need to realize that they can no longer teach, conceptualize, or evaluate their students' or residents' concerns about commercialism and lifestyle as if they are mere threats to professionalism. Instead, they need to acknowledge and address the complex reasons why the current generation considers these issues so important. This way, medical educators can provide students and residents the tools they need to uphold the professionalism promise they make to their patients and the society in which they live.

REFERENCES

Agar, M. (2003). Toward a qualitative epidemiology. *Qualitative Health Research*, 13(7), 974-986.

Aita, R., McIlvain, H., Susman, J., & Crabtree, B. (2003). Using metaphor as a qualitative analytic approach to understand complexity in primary care research. *Qualitative Health Research, 13(*10), 1419-31.

Anderson, R., Crabtree, B., Steele, D., & McDaniel, R. (2005). Case study research: The view from complexity science. *Qualitative Health Research*, 15(5), 669-685.

Anderson, R. & McDaniel, R. (2000). Managing health care organizations: Where professionalism meets complexity science. *Health Care Management Review, 25*(1), 83-92.

Axelrod, R. (1997). *The complexity of cooperation: Agent-based models of competition and collaboration.* Princeton, NJ: Princeton University Press.

Bak, P. (1999). *How nature works: The science of self-organized criticality.* New York, NY: Copernicus, Springer-Verlag, Inc.

Bar-Yam, Y. (1997). *Dynamics of complex systems.* Boulder, CO: Westview Press, Perseus Books Group.

Barabási, A. (2002). *Linked: The new science of networks.* Cambridge, MA: Perseus Publishing.

Bodenheimer T. (1999). The American health care system: Physicians and the changing medical marketplace. *New England Journal of Medicine, 340,* 584-588.

Brown, R. (1979). Rockefeller medicine men: Medicine and capitalism in America. Berkeley, CA: University of California Press.

Burrow, J. (1977). *Organized medicine in the progressive era: The move toward monopoly.* Baltimore, MD: Johns Hopkins University Press.

Byrne, D.S. (1998). *Complexity theory and the social sciences.* London: Routledge.

Caelleigh, A.S. (2001). The social contract. *Academic Medicine, 76,* 1174.

Capra, F. (1996). *The web of life.* New York, NY: Anchor Books Doubleday.

Capra, F. (2002). *The hidden connections: Integrating the biological, cognitive, and social dimensions of life into a science of sustainability.* NY: Doubleday.

Carr-Saunders, A., & Wilson, P. (1933/1964). *The professions.* London: F. Cass.

Castellani, B., & Castellani, J. (2003). Data mining: Qualitative analysis with health informatics data." *Qualitative Health Research, 13*(7), 1005-1018.

Castellani, B., Castellani, J., & Spray, S. (2003). Grounded neural networking: Modeling complex quantitative data. *Symbolic Interaction, 26*(4), 577-589.

Castellani, B., &. Hafferty, F. (forthcoming). *The sociology of complexity.*

Casti, J. (1999). The computer as laboratory: Toward a theory of complex adaptive systems. *Complexity, 4*(5), 12-14.

Cilliers, P. (1998). *Complexity and postmodernism: Understanding complex systems.* New York, NY: Routledge.

Coulehan, J., & Williams, P. (2003). Conflicting professional values in medical education. *Cambridge Quarterly of Healthcare Ethics, 12*(1), 7-20.

Coulehan, J., Williams, P., Van McCrary, S., Belling, C. (2003). The best lack all conviction: Biomedical ethics, professionalism, and social responsibility. *Cambridge Quarterly of Healthcare Ethics, 12*(1), 21-38.

Daniels N., Light, D., & Caplan, R. (1996). *Benchmarks of fairness for health care reform.* New York: Oxford University Press.

Farmer, P. (2003). *Pathologies of power: Health, human rights, and the new war on the poor.* Berkeley, CA: University of California Press.

Fox, E., Arnold, R.M., & Brody, B. (1995). Medical ethics education: Past, present, and future. *Academic Medicine, 70,* 761-769.

Freidson, E. (2001). *Professionalism: The third logic.* Chicago, IL: University of Chicago Press.

Freidson, E (1970a). *Professional dominance.* Chicago, IL: Aldine.

Friedson, E. (1970b). *Profession of medicine.* New York, NY: Dodd Mead.

Geyer, F., & van der Zouwen, J. (Eds.) (2001). *Sociocybernetics: Complexity, autopoiesis, and observation of social systems.* Westport, CT: Greenwood Publishing Group.

Gleick, J. (1987). *Chaos: Making a new science.* New York, NY: Penguin Books.

Hafferty, F. (2004) Toward the operationalization of professionalism: A commentary. *American Journal of Bioethics 4*(2), 28-32.

Hafferty, F. (2005). The elephant in medical professionalism's kitchen. *Academic Medicine.* (in press)

Hafferty, F., & Light, D. (1995). Professional dynamics and the changing nature of medical work. *Journal of Health and Social Behavior, 35(*Extra Issue), 132-153.

Hafferty F., & McKinlay J. (1993). *The changing medical profession: An international perspective.* New York: Oxford University Press.

Haug, M. (988) A re-examination of the hypothesis of physician deprofessionalization. *Milbank Quarterly, 66*(Supplement 2), 48-56.

Hilfiker, D. (2002). *Urban injustice: How ghettos happen.* NY: Seven Stories Press.

Holland, J. (1998). *Emergence: From chaos to order.* Cambridge, MA: Perseus Books.

Holland, John 1995. *Hidden order: How adaptation builds complexity.* Reading, MA: Addison-Wesley.

Hsia, D.C. (2001). Can joint negotiation restore physicians' professional autonomy? *Annals of Internal Medicine, 134,* 780-782.

Kauffman, S. (2000). *Investigations.* New York: Oxford University Press.

Klir, G.J. (2001). *Facets of systems science* (2nd ed.). New York, NY: Kluwer Academic/Plenum Publishers.

Lindorff, D. (1992). *Marketplace medicine: The rise of the for-profit hospital chains.* New York, NY: Bantam.

Lewis, S. (1925/1998). *Arrowsmith.* New York, NY: Penguin-Putnam Inc.

Luhmann, N. (1995). *Social systems: Outline of a general theory.* Stanford, CA: Stanford University Press.

Mandelbrot, B. (1983). *The fractal geometry of nature.* New York, NY: Freeman.

Maturana, H., & Varela, F. (1992). *The tree of knowledge: The biological roots of human understanding.* Boston, MA: Shambala.

McDaniel, R., Jordan, M.. & Fleeman, B. (2003). Surprise, surprise, surprise! A complexity science view of the unexpected. *Health Care Management Review, 28*(3), 266-278.

McGaghie, W., Mytko J., Brown, W., & Cameron, I. (2002). Altruism and compassion in the health professions: A search for clarity and precision. *Medical Teacher, 24,* 374-378.

McKinlay, J., & Arches, J. (1985). Toward the proletarianization of physicians. *International Journal of Health Services, 15*(2), 161-195.

McKinlay, J., & Stoeckle, J. (1988). Corporatization and the social transformation of doctoring. *International Journal of Health Services, 18*(2), 191-205.

Miller, W., McDaniel, R., Crabtree, B., & Stange, K. (2001). Practice jazz: Understanding variation in family practice using complexity science. *Journal of Family Practice, 50*(10), 872-878.

Rippe, J.M. (1999). *Lifestyle medicine.* Malden, MA: Blackwell Science

Schiedermayer, D., & McCarthy, D.J. (1995). Altruism, professions, decorum and greed: Perspectives on physician compensation. *Perspectives in Biology and Medicine, 38,* 238-253.

Schneider, C.E. (1998). *The practice of autonomy: Patients, doctors, and medical decisions.* New York; Oxford University Press.

Schwartz, R.W., Jarecky, R.K., Strodel, W.E., Haley, J.V., Young, B., & Griffen, W.O.J. (1989). Controllable lifestyle: A new factor in career choice by medical students. *Academic Medicine, 64,* 606-609.

Starr, P. (1982). *The social transformation of American medicine.* New York, NY: Harper Collins Basic Books.

Waitzkin, H. (1991). *The politics of medical encounters: How patients and doctors deal with social problems.* New Haven, CT: Yale University Press.

Waldrop, M. (1992). *Complexity: The emerging science at the edge of order and chaos.* New York, NY: Simon & Schuster.

Ward, M. (1999). *Virtual organisms: The startling world of artificial life.* New York, NY: St. Martin's Press.

Watts, D. (1999). *Small worlds: The dynamics of networks between order and randomness.* Princeton, NJ: Princeton University Press.

Wear, D., & Kuczewski, M. (2004). The professionalism movement: Can we pause? *American Journal of Bioethics, 4*(2), 1-10.

Wear, D., & Castellani, B. (2002). Motherhood and medicine: The experience of double consciousness. *Annals of Behavioral Science and Medicine Education,8*(2), 92-96.

Chapter 2

AN ANALYSIS OF THE DISCOURSE OF PROFESSIONALISM

Jamie L. Shirley and Stephen M. Padgett
University of Washington

INTRODUCTION

The field of medicine as a clinical profession is widely perceived to be under siege these days, though the perceived assaults come from a confusing combination of directions. Managed care organizations, government regulators, competing professional groups, "alternative and complementary" practitioners, vengeful lawyers, crusading political activists, unhappy consumers (formerly known as patients, and now unhappy for all sorts of reasons), and others attack from the outside. Meanwhile from within, the explosion of new medical information, the inability to clarify the roles of generalists and specialists, the growing concern about health disparities and the social determinants of health, the persistent inattention to prevention, the catastrophe of tens of millions who remain uninsured or underinsured—all of these crises (and any of us could name yet more) have made the clinical practice of medicine an uncertain and troubled occupation. This, in turn, has made basic medical education—the preparation of new practitioners—enormously challenging.

One response to the crises in medical practice and medical education has been a call for a "renewed professionalism." The American Board of Internal Medicine (ABIM, 1995), the Association of American Medical Colleges (AAMC, 1998), and other professional organizations and individual educators (e.g. Pellegrino, 2002) have issued calls for a return to the ideals at the moral core of the profession of medicine. The discussion, as it is most commonly framed, focuses primarily on inculcating in physicians a set of (not particularly controversial) virtues, such as altruism, duty, and integrity. These virtues have been widely criticized as too vague, and not surprisingly, some commentators have called for more precise, concrete, and measurable definitions (Connelly, 2003; Wear & Nixon, 2002).

The issues that underlie the recent calls for a renewed professionalism within medicine deserve focused attention, such as the concern for excellence in patient care, the appropriate regulation of practitioners, and the need to adequately serve community needs. However, we believe that the proposed approach is not an effective or useful response to the multiple crises in medical education. The problem is not just a matter of the ambiguity of the invoked virtues, but rather that efforts toward definitional precision and measurement rely on a mistaken view of language and of the relationship between language, social institutions, and practice. An even more fundamental problem is the effort to locate the solution to systemic problems of medical education and practice in the virtues of individual physicians.

We will argue that the "renewed professionalism" movement reflects deeply held (though confused) beliefs about the role and status of professions—what we will call "the discourse of professionalism." This discourse of the professionalism is powerful in part *because* of its ideological confusion; that is, its ambiguity works to unify and solidify social networks and interests, and to make that unity seem natural and inevitable. However, the organizing work of professionalism discourse has become increasingly untenable, and the tensions within this discourse—especially as it is used within medicine—are becoming more difficult to avoid. The discourse of medical professionalism is not likely to be salvageable through the "new professionalism" project. What is instead required is the more difficult (and politically charged) project of re-negotiating the social contract between physicians, communities, and other occupational groups.

This paper will begin with a discussion of two broad models of language, the conventional one of language as a symbolic or representational system, and an alternate one, in which language is seen as a social practice. We will then examine the social context within which the discourse of professionalism is enacted and the multiple purposes it serves. In particular, we will focus on the recent changes in social and cultural institutions and practices upon which medical professionalism depends and through which it occurs. Recent calls for a "new professionalism" tend to ignore those institutions and social changes (as well as the problematic aspects of the profession's claims to authority and power). As a result, the movement is limited in its ability to help physicians and educators cope with those changes and transform those institutions, or to help contemporary communities negotiate more effectively with the medical system to meet their own needs. Finally, we will address how the confluence of discourse theory and the rhetoric of virtue ethics offers the potential to see a more useful direction for the reform of medical education and medical professionalism.

AN ALTERNATIVE MODEL OF LANGUAGE

The conventional model of language presumes that language is referential and transparent. Language is held to be comprised of words, and these words are symbols that represent or refer to "things in the world." These things may be objects (a table), ideas (honesty), or activities (running), and for each, meaning is derived from the word's correspondence with its object. Additionally, this model assumes that we can reliably know to which objects the words refer. By this criterion, good language is that which allows one to see through it with a minimum of ambiguity to the objects it represents (Rorty, 1979).

By contrast, an alternative account calls attention to how languages function as social practices—not as names for public objects or private experiences, but as interactional events and social transactions. (While our account here is drawn largely from post-structuralism, there is a broad consensus among several contemporary philosophies of language, including Bakhtin [1984], Rorty [1979], Shotter [1993], Wittgenstein [1958], and others; see Stewart [1996] for an excellent overview.) Languages include words, of course, but these words point not toward objects but to other words, making a chain of signifiers. The linkages of this chain rely upon social processes and interactions to establish shared understandings about what the signifiers mean and, most importantly, how they are used (Allen & Hardin, 2001). Meanings are not fixed or predetermined, but they are limited by their contextual use; some interpretations are more strongly warranted than others. Thus, far from being transparent, these signifiers are taken to be understandable only when situated in a particular context (Gee, 1999). The ambiguity of terms such as "altruism," therefore, results not from a lack of definitional precision, but from the breakdown of the social practices and conventions that give it meaning by providing it shape, form, substance—and recognizability. The definition of altruism can be found in any dictionary, but knowing which behaviors and motives count as altruistic in a particular setting is a socio-cultural process and cannot be made fully explicit.

To emphasize the distinction between the notion of languages as "words and symbols" and the notion of languages as "social practices," we sometimes use the term *discourse* (Fairclough, 1992; Van Dijk, 1997). Discourses are composed of the practices and institutions of a particular social community, organized around a topic or activity, within a particular historical and cultural context—what people do, and how they do it. These social structures are largely responsible for the production of language, but are themselves contingent upon language to make them possible (Torfing, 1999). Various discourses are not just different words for the same things; instead, they help to construct *different* things, different ways of doing things, *and* different kinds of power.

This construction of difference is especially important in relation to the category of "personal experience." Discourses provide people with vocabularies through which to explain, to themselves and to each other, their actions and motivations in a way that is understandable (Mills, 1940). Accounts of experience are *always already* an interpretation of what has happened, and these accounts are subject to reinterpretation in the process of telling them to others. "What counts as experience is neither self-evident nor straightforward; it is always contested, and always therefore political" (Scott, 1992, p. 387). The production of language is always a communal enterprise, a series of negotiated exchanges with other speakers over time. Linguistic behavior only works when it is recognized by its audience as a certain kind of gesture (Gee, 1999). Through language, communities reproduce their structures, discipline their members, and enact social practices. Language is what we do, not merely how we talk about what we do (Shotter, 1993).

In addition to the elements of language as "social action" and as "vocabularies of motives and experience," three other elements of the post-representationalist approach to language are important for our purposes here. First, there is the multiplicity of available discourses. There is always more than one discursive option available to a speaker, more than one discourse circulating in society related to a particular topic. Second, there is the unevenness of this multiplicity. The full range of discourses potentially available at any one time and place are not equally available to all speakers, nor are they all equally powerful. The more hegemonic discourses (those produced by and reproducing powerful social institutions) tend to obscure competing discourses by making their own assumptions seem natural and unmarked, while discounting alternate constructions of the world or performances of identity (Nelson, 2001). In this way, discourses function as disciplining forces. That is, what it is possible to say or do is both enabled and constrained by the available linguistic and performative vocabulary (Torfing, 1999).

Finally, there is temporality and historicity. Discourses are not static, but dynamic and evolving. There is a constant negotiated process of reproduction, resistance, and creativity as communities work to determine meanings (Bakhtin, 1986). People can invoke discourses in ways that cut across or undermine the usual intent or pattern of a discourse. As they take up and use multiple discourses, the tensions among them may generate new or transformed discourses. In their turn, the practices and institutions they reinscribe are also transformed over time (Fairclough, 1992; Gee, 1999).

This view of language provides us with a way to look at the discourse of professionalism as a site of social action, a place where various communities are acting, and to locate those sites and communities in history. The discourse of professionalism helps to construct certain experiences and limit others, and is deeply entangled with particular institutions, power relationships, and cultural arrangements. It is a discourse that organizes relationships, provides plausible motives for people and causes for events, and is a site of struggle and change as those arrangements and institutions are adapted, resisted, and transformed.

The discourse of medical professionalism, then, includes these three aspects: *language* (the words used to describe and carry out the activities of medicine), *practices* (the behaviors that are entailed), and *institutions*. The language of professionalism includes the naming of virtues, such as altruism, duty, and excellence; it also describes who is included and who is excluded (e.g., physicians vs. "allied" professionals), the nature of the problems that profession is responsible for, and so on. The practices of professionalism are those which reinforce the assumptions of professionalism: the dyadic provider-patient relationships; the hierarchical naming of physicians, other health care providers, and patients; the expectation of unpredictable work hours (Lupton, 1994). When we refer to the institutions of professionalism, we are primarily referring to the social and cultural ones, the ideas rather than the buildings. Thus hospitals, for example, support professionalism not only in their physicality, but also in their ideological structures, which are designed around the work of physicians (Starr, 1982). Other institutions also participate in the discourse of professionalism, such as marriage and other gendered institutions, the authority of science, and academic medicine.

This understanding of the discourse of medical professionalism guides us away from efforts at definitional precision, away from asking what particular terms mean (or should mean.) Rather, we can ask, what does this language *do*? What are we using it for, and perhaps, what is it using *us* for? Why is it being taken up *now*, and by whom, and for what practical or political purposes?

For example, "excellence" is defined by the ABIM proposal as "the conscientious effort to exceed ordinary expectations" (ABIM, 1995, p. 6). Beyond the obvious questions of "by how much?" and "what is a 'conscientious effort'?" there is the thornier question of how the baseline "ordinary" expectations are established.   To what extent are those expectations determined by the physical resources available to the physician (for example, the lone physician in a rural hospital vs. an urban tertiary care center)?   Who has the power to determine those "ordinary" expectations—patients?   Other physicians?   The insurance company?

To understand how the discourse of professionalism works to accomplish these tasks, we need to situate the professions in a broader social and historical context. We specifically want to draw attention to the relationship between the *social structures* of the professions (especially the medical profession) and the *discourse* of professionalism—and in several areas, to notice the growing gaps between them, the ways that professionalism discourse is less able to effectively *make sense* of the contemporary practice of medicine.   (We mean the phrase "making sense" more literally than is usually implied—i.e., the *construction* of sense and meaning, the giving of order, form, and substance.)

THE DISCOURSE OF PROFESSIONALISM

There are four points about our understanding of professionalism that are most relevant for this discussion. The first is the idea that professions are rooted in a *social contract*, an agreement between the State and the members of the occupational group. The second is that this social contract is widely acknowledged to function poorly in a number of key aspects. The third is that the professions—like all social organizations—rely upon and are enacted through an interlocking set of institutions, including languages, cultural mores and expectations, and interpersonal relationships. The final point is that being a profession is neither an inherent attribute nor an objective characteristic of any particular occupation. Professionalism is not, in a sense, a status at all; it is a *claim* to a certain status, a claim that is more or less successful within a particular social context (Abbott, 1988; Park, 2004).   None of these points about professions is, by itself, very controversial. Taken together, however, and viewed through the prism of discourse theory, they provide insights about the challenges faced by those promoting education in medical professionalism.

The conventional description of the professions as operating under a social contract refers to the idea that society (via the State) grants professional groups a degree of autonomy in exchange for self-regulation. Professional self-regulation is the promise that the profession will establish and enforce standards of education and practice, and that incompetent or unethical practitioners will be disciplined, sanctioned, or excluded. This policy of self-regulation (with minimal interference from the State) is justified by the premise that professional groups are in the best position to evaluate and manage the conditions of practice for their own members.

This contract has a *collective* nature; it is a contract between all medical professionals and society. A physician's professional ethics are not personal virtues, values, or rules; rather, they are derived from her or his adherence to a set of group norms. This is important because it brings our attention back to the institutions, social practices, and cultural arrangements through which professionals operate.

In addition to the ideal of "self-regulation," two other concepts are crucial to this version of professionalism: (a) that professional practice is oriented toward the public good, rather than the self-interest of either individual or collective professionals, and (b) that there is a legitimating body of knowledge—the *science* of medicine or nursing, or legal knowledge— distinct from tradition, mere whim, or self-interest (Freidson, 1970; Moore, 1970).

Sociologists and historians have become increasingly skeptical of professional claims in all these areas (Abbott, 1988; Freidson, 1970, Starr, 1982). The ability or willingness of professional groups to regulate the practices of their members, the extent to which professions can put the public good above their collective self-interest, and even the solidity of the knowledge base on which professional practice allegedly rests—all of these have come to be seen as far more dubious and partial than professionalizing proponents would have us believe. For most sociologists and historians, professionalism—or more precisely the process of professionalization—is principally about the control of work, about who is allowed to do it (and who is not), the status of those practitioners, and the conditions under which the work is to be done.

The claims to professional status are efforts to control the conditions of work, training, compensation, and evaluation; they are claims to a cultural authority as well (Foley & Faircloth, 2003; Park, 2004). Medicine's power to define problems and assign solutions is not only the result of its control over conditions of work, but from its success in persuading the public that it speaks from a position of knowledge, compassion, and objectivity—that its voice is to be trusted, relied upon, accepted. Notwithstanding its current troubles, U.S. medicine has been extraordinarily successful in that persuasion (Starr, 1982). Professionalism in general and medical professionalism in particular are inextricably entangled with power and privilege, and have a long history of abuse of that power.

It is not necessary to take the sociological critiques of professionalism to mean that the medical community is engaged in deliberate deception. The trust developed between the professional and the client may be quite genuine, as might be the devotion to duty, the confidence in the science, the fellowship with one's colleagues. Discursive approaches to language provide a useful way to understand how this works. In this approach, the discourse is considered to be most effective when there is congruence among the ready-at-hand language, the dominant cultural traditions, the social practices of daily life, and the institutions in which physicians live and work. However, as the social context in which medicine is practiced changes, and the gaps between these elements widens, the unifying and solidifying work of this discourse is less effective, and the trust offered by the public becomes more tenuous and contested.

It is important to notice that the vocabulary of professionalism is deployed for different purposes with different audiences. For those within a particular occupational group, it is taken for granted that professionalism is a positive ideal, that it is connected with virtue (or some specific set of virtues), and that increasing professionalism means increasing the quality of practice. Professionalism in this context serves to promote confidence and authority, to identify some problems as important and others not, and to foster solidarity with other members.

When directed toward the public, by contrast, the discourse of professionalism is intended to foster trust in both the process and outcome of treatment. It is intended to reassure clients that practitioners are qualified, their judgments and advice are reliable and true, their services are necessary, and (not insignificantly) their fees justified. For both groups, professional discourse serves to obscure the power and privilege possessed by the practitioner group over the lives and interests of others, making that power and privilege seem natural, appropriate, and inevitable.

An example of the "naturalizing" power of this discourse is the way in which it institutionalizes (and makes invisible) a certain set of gendered relations. While the discourse of professionalism emphasizes the autonomy of practitioners, the practical work and lives of physicians are inextricably entangled with, and dependent upon, the work of others, primarily the work of women. In the public sphere, the work of physicians is dependent upon the work of less-prestigious occupations, such as nurses, social workers, physical and occupational therapists, and others, as well as an ensemble of even lower paid workers, such as housekeepers, nursing assistants, secretaries, and clerks. The labor of these workers is largely made invisible by the discourse of medical professionalism, through its exclusionary focus on the individual practitioner (Davies, 1996).

As an illuminating counter-example, we would note that the discourse of professionalism is more complicated when invoked by members of other health care occupations. For nurses and social workers, as an example, the power and privileges of professionalism are far more tenuous than for physicians (Melosh, 1982; Reverby, 1987). Both of these largely female groups, doing work that historically has been devalued or ignored, have always worked under conditions in which their work is constrained by institutions, and clearly entangled with the work of others (Abbott & Meerabeau, 1998). Claiming professional status thus works paradoxically, both to assert their right to the autonomy and status of other professional groups, and to call attention to the limits of those as markers of professionalism. Regardless of the efficacy of the claims to professional status by these groups, however, the increasing use of the discourse of professionalism by them has disrupted the credibility of medicine's claim to a uniquely privileged and autonomous practice. By making their own labor more visible, nurses, social workers, and those in other health care occupations have also made more visible the dependence on and interconnectedness of medicine to their work.

Medicine's dependence on a set of gendered relationships and social structures is equally important in the domestic or private sphere. At home, the conventional role of the physician relies on women's work as well, assuming the availability of a supportive spouse, childcare provider, and homemaker to enable the obligations of the professional calling. For physicians with children, in particular, the daily tasks such as playing with and reading to children, caring for them when they are sick, transporting them to extracurricular activities, and managing play-dates and homework have traditionally been done by mothers. Meanwhile, the preparation of meals, the maintenance of the home, and the nurturance of the social network have traditionally been done by wives (Cowen, 1983). Waiting at home for a repairman and waiting at home for a child after school are alike in that someone must *be* at home, not just intermittently, but day after day, night after night. The traditional wife and mother waits for the physician as well, providing a safe harbor, a warm dinner, a listening heart. This support has allowed physicians to maintain extended and unpredictable working hours, to cope with the emotional challenges of sickness and death, and to belong to a community outside the hospital and clinic—to have a life as well as a career. The supportive labor by others in the domestic sphere also, of course, allows the medical system to expect this kind of work schedule of individual physicians (Hochschild & Machung, 1989; Hochschild, 2003).

The profound, although incomplete, shifts in social roles for men and women over the last few decades, including the entrance of more women into the practice of medicine and more generally into the paid workforce, have interrupted these assumptions. Most obviously, women physicians are less likely to have a spouse who can manage their private lives while they focus on their professional roles. (The pool of potential wives for female surgical residents is remarkably small.) To some extent this is also true for men, who are increasingly likely to have spouses with their own careers, interests, and obligations outside the home. Male physicians are also more likely than in past generations to make participation in childcare and other familial obligations a priority.

In linguistic terms, we might say that these young physicians are caught between several powerful and competing social discourses, for example, one about parenting and the other about professionalism. The professionalism discourse emphasizes that the interests of the patient take priority over the self-interest of the physician. Meanwhile, the discourse of modern parenting instructs parents that the most valuable assets they can give their children are time and attention. (This emphasis on individual parenting is enforced by the lack of social resources, such as access to flexible childcare arrangements and part-time work schedules, and school schedules that presume a stay-at-home caregiver.) Both of these discourses highlight special obligations to people with dependency needs, but neither offers guidance as to how those obligations should be reconciled or combined. Other competing discourses include the contemporary emphasis on building emotional intimacy with one's partner, adequate "self-care," and creating "balance" between work, family, play, and personal meaning (Hafferty, 2003). All of these obligations pull away from a simple or straightforward application of altruism, fidelity, or public service.

In addition to the changes in gendered relations, there are changes in other institutions that surround and support medical professionalism. Patients approach their physicians with a broader (and sometimes contradictory) set of discourses available to them for negotiating the physician-patient relationship. Patients come to their appointments armed with information from the Internet and with directives from pharmaceutical companies to "Ask your physician!" Consumer groups urge patients to come with a list of questions, to take notes and "shop around," to be more skeptical of advice and more involved in decision-making. The growing discourses of patient rights, patient autonomy, and patient involvement all complicate the traditional role of physician as expert with privileged knowledge.

Some patients, however, never get to an appointment at all because a growing number of persons living in the U.S. are un- or under-insured. The virtue of fidelity can reasonably be understood and practiced with a single patient, but when faced with a caseload of patients, communities, populations, or society-at-large, the meaning of this principle is much less clear. The framing of the physician-patient relationship as a "dyad" makes it difficult to negotiate questions of wider social responsibilities, to take up questions of social policy, or even to make sense of the multiple demands on any given practitioner. When the medical profession has taken up the topic of nationalized health care (through the AMA and other professional organizations), it has repeatedly affirmed its commitment to this conservative notion of fidelity by opposing socialized medicine (Navarro, 1993; Rothman, 1994).

Meanwhile, the assumption of the professional's clinical autonomy is challenged by the changing structure of health care institutions and the financing of those institutions. Physicians are increasingly providing care as members of collaborative teams, and as salaried employees in large group practices. They share patients with specialists (both physician and non-physician), and relinquish care to hospitalists when their patients are institutionalized.

Indeed, physicians today are facing multiple forms of external review of their clinical practice. Although managed care organizations have been the most explicit about this evaluative process, all health care institutions are looking carefully at how resources are utilized, both capital and human. The question of clinical efficacy for a particular patient has been supplemented by questions of efficacy and cost-effectiveness for populations. What care should be provided, and by whom, and who should decide? How much attention should providers give to financial considerations in clinical decisions? How should we evaluate quality of care? Should the emphasis in medical practice be on standardization or individualization? The traditional discourse of professionalism provides little or no help on these issues.

The movement for evidence-based practice (EBP) is another form of external review that runs counter to the presumptive autonomy of the clinical practitioner (Tanenbaum, 1994). The EBP movement is particularly skeptical of the idea of "clinical judgment"—the idea that individual physicians are in the best position to know what is best for their individual patients. EBP proponents assert instead that individual practitioners are often wrong about what works, either because of various biases built into their memory of practice, or because they simply cannot keep up with the flood of new studies (Tanenbaum, 1999). While in some ways the EBP movement relies on traditional and even conservative ideas about science (for example in its preference for quantitative data from large, randomized, and highly standardized clinical trials), in other ways the EBP approach works to undermine the authority of the science of medicine. Any given recommendation is only "the best we know now" and could just as easily change tomorrow; in fact, the recent history of medical guidelines in several areas has demonstrated this instability to alarming proportions (e.g., hormone replacement therapy).

Though the discourse of professionalism has long been effective in covering over internal conflicts and bridging external tensions, it can no longer contain the contradictory changes occurring in society. Multiple competing discourses are increasingly challenging the hegemony of traditional medical professionalism, including consumerism, changing social roles for men and women, and systems-based approaches to quality-improvement and patient safety. In light of this analysis, recent calls for a renewed professionalism would seem to be an overly simplistic solution to a complex situation. The social pressures to which it is attempting to respond are too diverse to be contained by the old model.

Professionalism has always been a negotiation between the interests of professionals and those of the public. What has changed are both the perception of those interests and the context in which those negotiations occur. Health care is increasingly the work of teams and systems, not autonomous individuals or even single professions. Notions of the "public good" are in themselves more contested and uncertain. A host of social changes has shifted both the internal demographics of medical students and their expectations and options for the future. A renewed professionalism would need to take into account all these changes. Attempts to concretize professional virtues, and hold medical students accountable for them, have got the process exactly backwards. What we first need to do is re-negotiate the social practices on which those values rest, and re-configure the institutions that produce them.

As this discussion has shown, the discourse of medical professionalism depends on—and operates through—a set of interlocking institutional, cultural, political, and economic structures, structures which the discourse renders largely invisible. Those social systems are now in transition, however, and the tensions and contradictions in them are more apparent. Because of this, the discourse of professionalism no longer works and no longer makes sense, for it is increasingly unable to account for the lives and choices of its participants.

DISCOURSE AND VIRTUE ETHICS

By using the language of virtue, medical educators are acknowledging that this effort to revive professionalism is essentially an ethical project. Setting aside our skepticism about possible motives for this latest version, the project of developing virtues in novice practitioners has a venerable history, which has been recently reinvigorated (MacIntyre, 1984; Pellegrino & Thomasma, 1993). The effort to help members of the medical community become the right kind of people, to develop in them the moral character required to act appropriately, is a task undertaken with the ethical intent of ensuring that novice physicians will honor the social contract established between the profession and the public.

While derived from very different intellectual traditions, the *practical* work of virtue ethics shares much with discourse theory. Like virtue ethics, discourse theory suggests that moral activity is guided more by implicit cultural norms than by explicit rules, that we learn by doing, and that our ethical character is shaped by the community in which we live and act (McKinnon, 1999). All communities discipline their members, strive to make them become certain kinds of persons rather than others, and construct those choices as "natural." Virtue ethics and discourse theory understand the nature of action very differently, however. While discourse theory calls attention to the central role of language in establishing, communicating and enacting normative practices, virtue ethics presumes that behaviors arise from proper character. Character, though it can be enhanced through teaching, is an essential feature of an individual, and even the correct action cannot be considered virtuous unless it arises from this innate desire to do and be good (Aristotle, 1962).

What virtue ethics assumes, discourse theory makes explicit, and the professionalism project seems to have forgotten, is that for this discipline to be effective, there must be strong community consensus about the virtues being established. This consensus must be supported by everyday practices and by social institutions. The virtue ethics model presumes a fairly homogeneous community with clearly delineated roles and strong mentors, for the virtues are learned through the internalization of these roles, and through living out those roles in one's own life and work (Pellegrino, 2002).

This ideal of a stable community is clearly at odds with the pluralistic and fragmented nature of contemporary American society. Novice physicians (medical students and residents) are enmeshed in a variety of powerful social discourses, not only medical professionalism, and they (like all of us) are pulled in many directions in the construction of their identities, their values, and their practices (Good & DelVecchio Good, 1993). Within medical schools, the traditional hegemony of wealthy white males is eroding. The view of language outlined here would suggest that this discourse of professional virtues is not equally accessible to those who do not fit this demographic: women, minorities, and students from the working class, for example (More & Milligan, 1994; Beagen, 2001).

The social contract between physicians and society is a social system of rights, duties, and reciprocal relationships. Individual virtue is tied to community virtue in that physicians are (in this model) entitled to certain privileges and expectations in exchange for their service to the community. To the extent that physicians are no longer receiving the social power they desire and the society is not satisfied with the service they receive, it is a collective problem. It reflects a breakdown in reciprocity on both sides of the contract.

Virtue ethicists and discourse analysts would agree that it is not enough to give students words—the names of virtues—because words alone do not have meaning; they must be backed by practices. Even if we give students those practices, however, even if they have role models to teach them these practices, the practices have to make sense within (and make sense of) the institutional structures as they currently exist (both internal and external to health care). It is not enough to have faculty who can empathize with the struggles of a physician missing his daughter's soccer game in order to admit a patient; that is not developing virtue but rather using "altruism" to maintain a dysfunctional system. We must create ways of taking care of patients that also allow the taking care of children. Similarly, it is not enough for faculty mentors to rail against the intrusions of managed-care organizations into the patient-provider relationship without at the same time showing young physicians other ways of taking up the issues of distributive justice and the proper allocation of limited resources.

The effort to locate professionalism in individual physicians misses the collective nature of values and virtues, the ways they are fundamentally community-based practices. Virtues require community support, not only in the educational process, but also in the practical sense of institutions structured so as to make the exercise of those virtues possible. Language works by pointing toward knowledge to which we already collectively have access. We must be able to recognize and participate in embodied practices and institutions, or the words cannot have meaning. We need virtues that can inspire moral courage and right action, but more than lists of virtues, we need new *institutions* to support and embody such virtues.

CONCLUSIONS

Efforts to revive the discourse of professionalism within contemporary medical education and practice are therefore both misguided and unworkable. They are misguided because they are based on mistaken and unhelpful ideas about the way languages work. Language cannot be imposed from "out there," but must be negotiated in the context of daily practices and interactions. The work of making sense relies on the recognizability of the discourse for the people using it. These efforts are unworkable because they are trying to do too many different things under a single rubric. We cannot easily disentangle the "noble ideals" of professionalism from its more tawdry and self-serving components; we cannot simply extend the old arrangements that privileged a certain class to include a wider population; we cannot recreate the social conditions, public and private, that made both the privileges and the virtues meaningful and practical.

Continuing to use the language of professionalism without confronting the institutional and cultural infrastructure upon which it depends—and the changes that have occurred in those supporting structures, incomplete and uneven though they are—will only exacerbate the confusion and hostilities that characterize the current debate. What we need to do instead is both much harder and more ordinary. We must create institutions in which it is possible for medical trainees and practitioners to behave decently, to provide adequate care for their patients and to lead reasonable lives (with families, other interests, and enough sleep, for example). We must continue to re-negotiate the moral, political, and economic relationships and contracts among health care providers, patients, and communities. We must avoid the siren songs of nostalgia, sentimentalism, and cynicism. We must find language to express and inspire moral courage and integrity without requiring either heroic self-sacrifice or the invisible sacrifice of others.

A more nuanced view of the relationships among language, experience, social practices, and institutions, will help us here, as will a humbler view of medical practice. The challenges of medical education and practice have some particular characteristics, but many of them are shared by other health practitioners, by other occupations, and by all working people. We can all appreciate the difficulties of blending careers and families, of making room both for the work and the people one loves, for those are the difficulties of many working people. We urge physicians and medical educators to look at those difficulties as *public* problems, needing public solutions, and not as failures of individuals who are insufficiently dedicated. The problems of medicine cannot be addressed at the level of the individual practitioner, nor even at the level of the individual discipline. Physicians, with other health care workers, need to engage with their communities in a political process to decide how health care will be provided, including by and for whom. The social nature of discourse refocuses our attention on the needs and desires of the practitioners, of the various involved communities, and especially, on the negotiated nature of the moral agreement between them.

REFERENCES

Allen, D., & Hardin, P. K. (2001). Discourse analysis and the epidemiology of meaning. *Nursing Philosophy, 2,* 163-176.

Abbott, A. D. (1988). *The system of professions: An essay on the division of expert labor.* Chicago, IL: University of Chicago Press.

Abbott, P., & Meerabeau, L. (Eds.). (1998). *The sociology of the caring professions* (2nd ed.). London: UCL Press.

American Board of Internal Medicine. (1995). *Project professionalism.* Retrieved May 1, 2005 from the ABIM website: http://www.abim.org/pdf/profess.pdf.

Aristotle. (1962). *Nicomachean ethics* (M. Ostwald, Trans.). Indianapolis, IN: Bobbs-Merrill.

Association of American Medical Colleges. (1998). *Learning objectives for medical student education: Guidelines for medical schools, report 1.* Retrieved June 1, 2005 from the AAMC website: http://www.aamc.org/meded/msop/msop1.pdf

Bakhtin, M. M. (1986). *Speech genres and other late essays* (V.W. McGee, Trans; C. Emerson & M. Holquist, Eds.). Austin, TX: University of Texas Press.

Beagan, B. (2001). Micro inequities and everyday inequalities: "Race," gender, sexuality and class in medical school. *Canadian Journal of Sociology, 26*(4), 583-610.

Connelly, J. E. (2003). The other side of professionalism: Physician-to-physician. *Cambridge Quarterly of Health care Ethics, 12*(2), 178-183.

Cowen, R. S. (1983). *More work for mother: The ironies of household technology from the open hearth to the microwave.* New York: Basic Books.

Davies, C. (1996). The sociology of professions and the profession of gender. *Sociology, 30*(4), 661-678.

Fairclough, N. (1992). *Discourse and social change.* Cambridge: Polity Press.

Foley, L., & Faircloth, C. A. (2003). Medicine as discursive resource: Legitimation in the work narratives of midwives. *Sociology of Health and Illness, 25*(2), 165-184.

Freidson, E. (1970). *Professional dominance: The social structure of medical care.* New York: Atherton Press.

Gee, J. P. (1999). *An introduction to discourse analysis: Theory and method.* London: Routledge.

Good B. J., & DelVecchio Good, M. J. (1993). Learning medicine: The construction of medical knowledge at Harvard Medical School. In S. Lindenbaum and M. Locke, (Eds.), *Knowledge, power, and practice: The anthropology of medicine and everyday life.* Berkeley, CA: University of California Press.

Hafferty, F, (2003). Finding soul in a "medical profession of one." *Journal of Health Politics, Policy and Law, 28* (1), 133-158.

Hochschild, A.R., & Machung, A. (1989). *The second shift: Working parents and the revolution at home.* New York: Viking.

Hochschild, A. R. (2003). *The commercialization of intimate life: Notes from home and work.* Berkeley, CA: University of California Press.

Lupton, D. (1994). *Medicine as culture: Illness, disease, and the body in Western society.* Thousand Oaks, CA: Sage.

MacIntyre, A. (1984). *After virtue* (2nd Edition). Notre Dame, IN: University of Notre Dame Press.

McKinnon, C. (1999). *Character, virtue theories, and the vices.* Peterborough, Ontario: Broadview Press.

Melosh, B. (1982). *The physicians hand: Work culture and conflict in American nursing.* Philadelphia, PA: Temple University Press.

Mills, C. W. (1940). Situated actions and vocabularies of motive. *American Sociological Review, 5,* 904-913.

More, E.S., & Milligan, M. A. (Eds.). (1994). *The empathic practitioner: Empathy, gender, and medicine.* New Brunswick, NJ: Rutgers University Press.

Moore, W. E. (1970). *The professions: Roles and rules.* New York: Russell Sage Foundation.

Navarro, V. (1993). *Dangerous to your health: Capitalism in health care.* New York: Monthly Review Press.

Nelson, H. L. (2001). *Damaged identities, narrative repair.* Ithaca, NY: Cornell University Press.

Park, D.W. (2004). The couch and the clinic: The cultural authority of popular psychiatry and psychoanalysis. *Cultural Studies, 18*(1), 109-133.

Pellegrino, E. D. (2002). Professionalism, profession and the virtues of the good physician. *Mount Sinai Journal of Medicine, 69*(6), 378-384.

Pellegrino, E. D., & Thomasma, D. C. (1993). *Virtues in medical practice.* Oxford: Oxford University Press.

Reverby, S.M. (1987). *Ordered to care: The dilemma of American nursing, 1850-1945.* New York: Cambridge University Press.

Rorty, R. (1979). *Philosophy and the mirror of nature.* Princeton, NJ: Princeton University Press.

Rothman, D. J. (1994). A century of failure: Class barriers to reform. In J. A. Morone & G. S. Belkin, (Eds.), *The politics of health care reform: Lessons from the past, prospects for the future* (pp. 11-25). Durham, NC: Duke University Press.

Scott, J. (1992). Experience. In J. Butler & J. Scott (Eds.), *Feminists theorizing the political.* New York: Routledge.

Shotter, J. (1993). *Conversational realities: Constructing life through language.* Thousand Oaks, CA: Sage Publications.

Starr, P. (1982). *The social transformation of American medicine.* New York: Basic Books.

Stewart, J. (Ed.). (1996). *Beyond the symbol model.* Albany, NY: SUNY Press.

Tanenbaum, S. J. (1994). Knowing and acting in medical practice: The epistemological politics of outcomes research. *Journal of Health Politics, Policy and Law, 19*(1), 27-44.

Tanenbaum, S. J. (1999). Evidence and expertise: The challenge of the outcomes movement to medical professionalism. *Academic Medicine, 74*(7), 757-763.

Torfing, J. (1999). *New theories of discourse: Laclau, Mouffe and Zizek.* Oxford: Blackwell.

Van Dijk, T.A . (Ed.). (1997). *Discourse as social interaction.* Thousand Oaks, CA: Sage Publications.

Wear, D., & Nixon, L. L. (2002). Literary inquiry and professional development in medicine: Against abstractions. *Perspectives in Biology and Medicine, 45*(1), 104-124.

Wittgenstein, L. (1958). *Philosophical investigations* (3rd ed., G.E.M. Anscombe, Trans.). New York: Macmillan.

Chapter 3

PROFESSIONALISM
Curriculum Goals and Meeting Their Challenges

David J. Doukas
University of Louisville

The role of regulation, oversight, assessment, and compliance has been an under-recognized aspect of professionalism and medical ethics education in both medical school and residency. Medical educators need to appreciate the potential impact of recent mandates for professionalism by the Liaison Committee on Medical Education (LCME, 2004) and the Accreditation Council for Graduate Medical Education (ACGME, 1999). Professionalism is now a necessary and required part of medical student and house officer education. The concept of professionalism put forward by these organizations has been within the rubric of medical ethics, medical humanism, competency, and sound physician-patient communication. So, what do the ACGME and LCME require? Medical educators as well as learners need to understand what this joint framework of professionalism is and how it is to be taught and evaluated.

This chapter will discuss these organizations' criteria of accreditation in professionalism and examine their potential impact on the field of medicine. The particular impact in medical humanities education may be a significant byproduct of these curricular efforts. As a means to put these criteria into action, this chapter will present a model code of professionalism for medical students, residents, and their teachers. This code allows the medical learner to acknowledge openly and bear witness, with their professors, that they will uphold specific and implicit moral precepts in their educational apprenticeship that their professors will teach and role model to them. But, how can the content for this code be taught? How will success of this effort be measured? These considerations will be discussed in turn.

WHAT IS IT TO BE A PROFESSIONAL?

The professional binds oneself to a code of values and to each other in the profession, and promises to maintain one's skills and knowledge-based competence and profess the integrity of the set of skills and values for the practice of the profession. Furthermore, the professional is bound by a societal covenant to those he or she has been entrusted (Pellegrino & Thomasma, 1988; Ozar, 1995).

These concepts sound lofty, so why would anyone doubt the intent of those inclined to engage in a profession? We concern ourselves with professionalism of late due to the battering of the medical professionalism in the lay media that has occurred over the past 40 years. Medical care in the United States has changed in these past four decades from a predominantly fee-for-service mode (criticized as prone to abuse and avarice by the physicians) to managed care (criticized as being likewise ethically lapsed for the same reasons), tainted by the emergence of an overt two-tiered medical system (with all of its inherent injustice and the lack of practitioners willing to right this wrong). The practitioners of the medical arts have been pilloried in the lay media as self-interested, callous, unfeeling, and running from our societal obligations to care for the ill and poor of society. Further, medical error has been ascribed to lack of physician competence and/or sleep, with a remedy suggesting that professionalism would rectify these wrongs (Cassel, 2002).

It is no small wonder that organized medicine and its educational infrastructure has recoiled at these public perceptions. While it is intuitive that physicians should be trained in both the science and art of medicine, the past century has seen far more attention in medical education curriculum time to the science, rather than the art. This process may have been accelerated by the specialization of medicine, whereby more emphasis is on uses of technology rather than on how the physician interacts with the patient, the potential recipient of this technology.

The interest in professionalism was provoked in part by several public episodes where health care and ethics intersected. Whether it is due to the Nuremberg doctors' trials, the Tuskegee experiment, the Willowbrook scandal, or the Cruzan or Schiavo cases, medicine has been challenged by its inherent imbalance of art and science (Jonsen, 1999). During the past thirty years since the birth of modern bioethics, increased efforts have been made in teaching ethical theory to medical students (Lehmann, Kasoff, Koch, & Federman, 2004). Most efforts have focused on the pre-clinical phase of medical school, prior to the hands-on learning and interaction of patient interaction. While a helpful start, this effort alone is not the hoped-for end product of professionalism educational efforts. Articulating deontological arguments are, for example, but a means to start internal and group discussion of the ethical duties one has in practice.

Moral reflection and analysis is the stage beyond memorization of bioethical principles that requires working through ethical dilemmas. This process can occur in both the preclinical and clinical settings regarding patient-related cases and problems. Such interactions can be on a one-on-one or small group setting and now occur in many medical educational settings today. Regardless, reflection through analysis tests the physician-in-training to learn, and then use, a moral framework to work through an ethical problem. However, knowledge and analyses together are still not the end product sought in the quest for professionalism. The ability for a doctor to opine on a case, whether in real-time or from an ethics casebook, does not necessarily translate into the skills, attitudes, and behaviors that will promote humane and ethical conduct when she or he is working with patients and other health professionals.

Professionalism ultimately requires an end product of the demonstration of an understanding of moral skills and analysis through observable behavior (Surdyk, 2003). In the "see-one, do-one" world of medicine, one cannot hope for this to be a "procedure" seen once in others and then mastered. Professional conduct requires ongoing role modeling of those practitioners who are prime examples of their profession (Hatem, 2003; Kenny, Mann, & MacLeod, 2003). This is a very long row to hoe in medical education where the vast majority of educational venues depend on memorization of facts and regurgitation of the same on rote memorization tests. No, this facet of education is far more labor intensive for the teachers and other observers, as it requires observed interactions of medical learners with all forms of medical personnel and the patients they serve. It is evident that the outcome-based triad of knowledge, analysis, and behavior is the sought-after goal of the ACGME and LCME in the attainment of professionalism.

One glaring omission stands out in this educational discourse: What is it that we ask the physician-in-training to profess? What are medical learners expected to know regarding professionalism? How will they gain analytic skills in this process? How will medical learners incorporate those values and translate them into attitudes and behaviors that we require of the medical professional? How will we measure the attainment of these professional precepts and behaviors?

We do not want professionalism to be a lowest common denominator of conduct. (Past examples of learner assessment have included handwriting skills in charts and unkempt white coats.) We also know that little data supports the premise that there is moral development in house officers, for ethical erosion has been documented during training (Patenaude, Niyonsenga, & Fafard, 2003). The acculturation process could potentially transform the idyllic medical student into an attending physician with less, rather than more, moral sensitivity, analytic skills, and behavior. Clearly, this cynical end product is not the desired result of medical education. Given the concerns regarding error (as well as trust in patient care) by the Institute of Medicine, coupled with an increased concern regarding outcomes-based education, something clearly had to give—and give it did (Kohn, Corrigan, & Donaldson, 1999).

While such groups as the American Medical Association and the American College of Physicians regarded professionalism as a relevant essential precept, these doctrinal attempts by themselves could not move the educational state of the art of medical professionalism (Council on Ethical and Judicial Affairs, 2001; Medical Professionalism Project Members, 2002). What was needed was an articulation of what was expected in professional knowledge and conduct.

ENTER THE ACGME

The Accreditation Council of Graduate Medical Education (ACGME) precipitated this educational shift. The ACGME promulgated a set of guidelines of resident knowledge and behaviors called the General Competencies in 1999. The ACGME has the ability to shift the educational landscape so radically because their accreditation site visits to residency programs allow for full continued federal funding of these training programs. In short, their evaluation has enormous weight.

As identified by this author in 2003, almost two thirds of the six General Competencies are related to humanism, ethics, and professionalism (Doukas, 2003). While there is a Professionalism Competency specifically articulated, there are aspects of professionalism riddled throughout the General Competencies. In the Professionalism section, there is recognition of the need to learn and demonstrate both ethical principles and ethical virtues. Specific tasks are set out as well, such as confidentiality, informed consent, and cultural sensitivity.

Professionalism is also present elsewhere in the document, such as in the Patient Care, Interpersonal Communication Skills, and System-Based Practice Competencies. These sections call for humanistic skills of physician-patient relationships (with a need for boundary setting) as well as sound intra-professional relationships. Further, the place of the learner within a large, complex health system must be learned concurrently with the mandate of patient advocacy.

The General Competencies are relevant as leverage to house officer training programs to teach fundamental ethical precepts and then measure outcomes through behavior. The recommended ACGME Toolbox depends little on rote verbal or written testing either in person or online. Instead, the main educational thrust is on demonstrated behavior via small group discussion, standardized patients, OSCE exams and 360° evaluations of actual clinical performance.

By 2007, residency training programs are expected to have in place a system-wide General Competencies response (and currently are expected to be well along the road in development). An informal survey by this author of many residency programs reveals that most programs are aware of the General Competencies but few have developed a coherent response to them. Attempts to catalog resident professionalism curricula nationwide as well as a model curriculum in ethics and humanities has been undertaken by the American Society for Bioethics and Humanities (ASBH, 2005).

Site visitors have yet to evaluate professionalism as a component of education. Their timeline for implementation is over these next twenty-four months. Further, as ACGME requires outcomes data to improve individual and overall program performance, one wonders how residency programs can meet this mandate anytime soon. Given the premise of data equals medical education funding and improved safety, one might wonder: What is holding up progress?

THE LCME TETHER: SPURRING PROGRESS

In the past year, another pivotal aspect of education evaluation and professionalism has been added that will likely further the ACGME professionalism mandate. In 2004, the Liaison Committee on Medical Education (LCME) recently updated its accreditation standards for all medical schools (LCME, 2004). The LCME, which performs voluntary peer-review of North American medical schools, made an important change to its accreditation standards by tethering their goals in professionalism to those of the ACGME with the statement, "The objectives and their associated outcomes must address the extent to which students have progressed in developing the competencies that the profession and the public expect of a physician." Clearly, this linkage reveals that medical students are to be primed for their mission of engaging in professionalism education in their residencies.

As a prefatory section of the accreditations requirements for the schools themselves, the LCME sets out premedical requirements in section MS-1, stating that "students preparing to study medicine should acquire a broad education, including the humanities and social sciences. . . . General education that includes the social sciences, history, arts, and languages is increasingly important for the development of physician competencies outside of the scientific knowledge domain." While this concept has been circulated and promoted to pre-medical students for decades as contributing to well roundedness, few schools have implemented this "should" statement as a pre-condition for admission. The statement is attempting to encourage a balance of arts and science, and time will tell how medical schools will respond to this mandate.

In the educational requirement of medical schools, each school "must teach medical ethics and human values, and require its students to exhibit scrupulous ethical principles in caring for patients, and in relating to patients' families and to others involved in patient care" (ED-23). This effort requires not only coursework, then, but also evaluation of displayed behavior. Indeed, medical schools must establish a system for the evaluation of student achievement . . . [that] . . . should measure not only retention of factual knowledge, but also development of the skills, behaviors, and attitudes needed in subsequent medical training and practice, and the ability to use data appropriately for solving problems commonly encountered in medical practice (ED-26).

Observed behavior is therefore required as the student becomes more involved in patient care, with appropriate evaluative criteria to assess professional conduct. That is, "there must be ongoing assessment that assures students have acquired and can demonstrate on direct observation the core clinical skills, behaviors, and attitudes that have been specified in the school's educational objectives" (ED-27). This evaluation would then serve as a trip-wire for possible ethical breaches, and allow for addressing the student's shortcomings through remediation (Murden, Way, Hudson, & Westman, 2004).

Fundamental precepts of respect, honesty, and integrity are specifically set out as examples of ethical principles, but it is by no means an all-inclusive list. Noting that there is wide latitude on what each school deems "ethical behavior," the LCME then promotes a system of evaluating "skills, behaviors, and attitudes" that each student will need in their future development as a physician.

CONJOINED GOALS

What is the anticipated goal of the combined LCME-ACGME accreditation standards regarding professionalism? Ideally, all medical schools and residency programs would see the ongoing professional development of the physician-in-training as wholly embedded within their educational mandate. What is it we are to teach? Should we follow the letter of the accreditation guidelines using a minimalist interpretation? One would hope not. A more pragmatic operational view holds that the LCME purposefully set the stage for residency-based professionalism that will follow. ACGME then provides a detailed learning and evaluation experience in humanism, ethics, and professionalism. Such curricular integration thereby requires medical schools and residency programs to teach fundamental knowledge and skills to enable the health professional to be able to profess "professional" values and then behave in a way that exemplifies them.

But what exactly do the LCME and ACGME accreditation standards on professionalism say to us and our students? Surely, it is far more than "be professional." These two organizations have made explicit criteria that medical schools and residency programs must meet to be accredited and funded. While these educational goals are explicit to these educational programs, they are still quite opaque to the intended learners. How can students who frame their success in terms of basic science board exam scores appreciate what it is to be professional? If the goals, objectives, and measures of success are hidden from the learners, how can they ever hope to meet our, and their own, expectations?

We cannot expect that the learner will infer something that is currently just implied. A curriculum that hopes to convey concepts of humanism, ethics, and professionalism in a "hidden" manner runs the risk of remaining concealed entirely from the medical learner. Physicians-in-training are entitled to an explicit set of professional expectations in their knowledge and behavior. The medical learner needs a means by which to measure her performance and development, while also justifying the departure from her otherwise full bioscience curriculum. Essentially, students and residents need to understand that these "non-science" issues are on the test—both the National Boards (USMLE) and the everyday "test" of medical professionalism in their future, i.e., their professional life.

Any articulation of professionalism should allow the learner to know her professional goals, give her the means to meet them, and very importantly, clarify a set of shared values to profess. Such an articulation would allow the medical learner to engage in reflection on the moral standards being laid out.

The medical learner could then conceptualize her goals of knowledge and understanding, and put their corresponding behavioral ideals into practice.

The ACGME and LCME accreditation standards for professionalism are not all-inclusive of every humanistic, ethical, and professional ideal, and this author has taken ACGME to task on this very point (Doukas, 2003). However, it is feasible to read these standards and articulate a realistic set of values and behavioral goals that a physician-in-training can understand and put into action. These values listed below are not a confabulation of this author, but rather a synthesis of the LCME and ACGME values that are articulated in the accreditation documents regarding professionalism. This code articulates what physicians-in-training may strive for in their understanding and conduct. What follows is a melding together of the professionalism goals of the two accreditation documents into a single coherent code of professionalism to which a medical student or resident could then profess.

AN EDUCATIONAL CODE OF PROFESSIONALISM

I will strive for excellence in acquiring, maintaining, and displaying those areas of biomedical, social, and humanistic knowledge, skills, behaviors, and attitudes that enable me to care for my patient and be respectful of my patient's family, my colleagues, and my teachers.

I commit myself to the ethical principles and virtues of medicine. I will maintain a therapeutic and ethically sound interpersonal relationship with my patient and, as permitted by my patient, with the patient's family. I will hold information confidential as ethically and legally prescribed. I will be respectful of my patient and acknowledge the values and preferences of my patient in making health care decisions. I will be honest in my interactions and thereby facilitate the informed consent of my patient, including allowing my patient to withhold or withdraw treatment.

I will be a compassionate practitioner who will be caring in demeanor. I will be respectful of my patient in delivering health education, and of the options in improving health, or palliating discomfort. I will be respectful and sensitive to my patient's culture, belief systems, age, gender, and disabilities in their care. I will endeavor to address the total medical needs of my patient and appreciate the effects that social and cultural circumstances have on health care.

I will use medical information and investigations in a prudent and evidence-based manner when treating my patient. I will endeavor to apply knowledge systematically gained from the care of many patients and apply it to the patient before me, as well as in teaching other medical professionals. I will practice cost-effective care to treat my patient and I understand that my patient and I are part of a larger health care system. I will strive to be prudent in allocating resources in a way that does not compromise quality of care to my patient.

I will be my patient's advocate in his receiving quality care and help negotiate the complex system of health care. I will be an agent of change for my patient's betterment, and work effectively with other health professionals and managers to improve the health care of my patient. I will exhibit ethically sound business practices and demonstrate integrity in the care of my patient. I will not allow self-interest to jeopardize the care of my patient.

I will be entrusted to maintain all of these precepts and I will not condone their violation in my conduct or by other health professionals or those in training.

Deciphering the Code of Professionalism

This code of professionalism is intended to serve as a template for education, reflection, and action for the physician-in-training. As such, it sets out to encourage a knowledge-analysis-behavior framework to which both the institution and learner will be held accountable, as called on by both the ACGME and LCME accreditation standards. The knowledge to be learned is an understanding of those duties and aspects of character that enable a physician to be a sound professional. The behavior encouraged is an actualization of this knowledge with inculcated attitudes that epitomize these duties and virtues.

This code is a willing commitment to the humanistic, ethical, and professional values required of both learners and teachers. As these values are prescribed by both accreditation organizations, it is reasonable and justified that any medical student or resident in an accredited medical school or residency be able to profess the values that their institutions are mandated to teach. Contrariwise, medical institutions would be hard pressed to refuse to condone that these values be accepted as a code, as they must include them in their site visit documentation. These values are gathering points— one is hesitant to say consensus points—in humanism, ethics, and professionalism in contemporary medical education efforts of medical learners. Rather than attempt a comprehensive list of all medico-ethics-legal potential precepts and interactions, this code distills the essentials of the physician-patient professional interaction into those areas where most practitioners could agree, as currently articulated by ACGME and LCME.

The first sentence is an appeal to not only competence but also the striving for excellence in knowledge and skills. A critical part of the medical practitioner is the understanding that knowledge is a well that must be constantly drawn from in one's everlasting commitment to life-long learning. Of note, this appeal is not a narrow biomedical construct, but applies widely to areas of medicine, social discourse, and humanism. Further, this appeal goes beyond knowledge to the attainment of skills that will allow the learner to use that knowledge, and exhibit behaviors and attitudes that will demonstrate how such knowledge has become practice.

The code's commitment to the ethical principles and virtues of medicine makes clear that commitment to both duties and those aspects of personal character that facilitate sound health care will be learned and practiced (Pellegrino & Thomasma, 1993). Such commitment cannot be made in an open-ended, vague fashion. Hence, those duties (e.g., respect for persons) and virtues (e.g., compassion) that are explicitly identified by both LCME and ACGME are likewise articulated specifically. The bedrock of the medical encounter is an ethical and therapeutic relationship with the patient. This relationship has context and boundaries. Often, the patient will desire family-based involvement in their care. The family can and should be part of this relationship when the competent adult patient allows it. The involved parties can then define parameters of such a relationship, such as in the use of the family covenant (Doukas, 1991).

Confidentiality, a hallmark of this relationship, is defined as an ethical duty, with an understanding that harm to third parties (e.g. in infectious disease or threats of physical harm) are compelling reasons for breaching such confidences of medical information. The next statement asserts that respect is to be paid to the values and preferences of one's patient. This respect for persons is predicated on truthfulness to one's patient. Also, it follows that disclosure and respect for persons obliges the health professional to facilitate the process of the patient's informed consent. Such respect includes decisions to withhold or withdraw treatment, even if it may end the patient's life.

The following paragraph opens with a commitment to compassion in the care of patients. This virtue urges sensitivity in educating patients. The sought outcome is to heal and if unable to heal, to at least palliate one's patient from discomfort. Of particular importance, the learner is to recognize the need to be receptive and responsive to those of diverse backgrounds and infirmities. The code also promotes a comprehensive approach to patient care, while also being understanding of the socio-cultural context of health care for the patient.

The next paragraph opens with an appeal to the virtue termed *therapeutic parsimony* (Pellegrino & Thomasma, 1993). It is an appeal to neither practice defensively nor intuitively without evidence. Sound evidence-based medicine is an essential part of both beneficence and justice, as the physician should practice in those ways that help more than harm, and not spend frivolously on work-ups.

The systematic use of knowledge takes medical information writ large into the context of the individual patient-physician relationship. In turn, the physician sees his or her own role as a small player in a large stage. It also entreats the education of other physicians in the use of such knowledge. Cost effectiveness helps that whole system, but prudence in justice-based allocation does not mean their patient must suffer. Quality health care to one's own patient is sought in a fashion that does not jeopardize global-budgets.

The subsequent paragraph begins by reinforcing the duty of patient advocacy, particularly given the complexities of the health care system. This code asks of the physician to serve as a change agent for the individual patient as well as for the health care system. Of particular importance to one's future in the profession, sound business ethics are promised. Fraudulent behavior, deception, and "gaming the system" are not condoned. Further, self-effacement is a virtue appealed to, in which self-interest is set aside for the patient's benefit.

In its conclusion, the physician-in-training promises to adhere to this code. This promise of the medical learner and teacher is part of the fabric of the social covenant between physician and society. Given the educational foundation of the LCME and ACGME, it is the expectation that each institution will require the teaching of these precepts and each learner will adhere to them. Essential to this promise is the explicit pledge that any person who makes this promise must be held to it in order to be considered a professional. This code encourages honor and self-discipline among physicians to safeguard both patients and the integrity of the profession. It safeguards the profession by promising that practitioners will not condone inappropriate conduct, illegal behavior, or observed acts of malpractice.

Professing Professionalism

This code of professionalism would be best served by professing it repeatedly during the education of the physician-in-training. One method that may be helpful is to have a public reading upon the beginning of medical school. This reading could be during one of the many white coat ceremonies that now occur in medical schools across the country (Cohn & Lie, 2002). This reading would present the student with an open, public declaration that he or she is committed to professional conduct. This oath could be in addition to or instead of other ancient or modern oaths that have been used. Other mile markers of education when the code could be publicly professed include the transition into clinical clerkships and/or graduation from medical school. Similarly, this code could be professed upon entry into the residency, and on graduation from it.

Just as medical students and residents could profess this code, the teachers and physicians who engage in medical student and residency education should likewise profess these same precepts with their learners openly. Whether recited at a white coat ceremony or graduation, the code should be part of the culture of medical education for both medical learner and teacher. The professionalism code promotes its moral weight through the reciprocity of binding together student and teacher, and binding both of them to society.

The incorporation of this educational code repeatedly would serve two functions. First, the medical learner promises to the educational institution and medical profession that these expectations of knowledge and conduct will be acknowledged, acquired, and exemplified. Second, it is a promise of patient-centered behavior (i.e., the long sought outcome) that will then be assessed by the criteria laid out above. The code therefore reinforces what many consider implicit in medical education by making it explicit. This code closes the circle of accreditation body to educational program expectations of professionalism by making the student *part* of the pedagogical covenant.

Reciting a code is one thing, though, while implementing it is quite another. The reading of a code does not make it happen, just as the vocalization of a promise does not fulfill it. Medical schools and residency programs *must* meet LCME and ACGME mandates on professionalism, as these mandates have the moral and monetary weight to require education, quite unlike any other current code. The code is intended to put into action the promise made by these schools and programs to accreditation organizations by making this mandate clear, and by having them held accountable by their learners, not unlike the promise of a mentor to a protégé to provide education, training and support.

Medical schools and residency programs have widely varying degrees of programs in humanism, ethics, and/or professionalism. Some schools have developed their own codes of conduct, or have asked their students to innovate their own *de novo* (Fresa-Dillon, Cuzzolino, & Veit, 2004). What differentiates this code from others is that it makes the educational mandates of ACGME and LCME education clearly explicit and closes the circle of medical pedagogy (through the involvement of the learners) as a moral contract of professional education. Now, is the proposed code the be-all, end-all, of what such a code for medical learners would look like? Past argument might suggest that more conversation with teachers and learners would likely improve the comprehensiveness of the code (Doukas, 2003). Be that as it may, the proposed code allows for both a promise to fulfill the educational mandates, and a measuring stick of expectation of teachers should instruct and role model and what learners should incorporate and exemplify.

Teaching Professionalism

Translating the precepts of this code into action will be a formidable challenge for medical schools and residency programs. Humanism, ethics, and professionalism are, by their nature, a broad thematic thrust of what is to be a medical professional. Teaching these core precepts of professionalism (by instruction and role modeling) is far too important to the comportment of the physician to be squandered in some "orphan topic" bin of miscellaneous doctoring courses in medical school. Often times, though, this is precisely what happens. Physician communication skills and medical ethics are often foisted upon students with other (seemingly) random topics, thus rendering their importance moot in the mind of the medical learner (Coulehan & Williams, 2003).

Curriculum time equals respect and recognition. Similarly, being a recognized course or sub-course with its own grading conveys to students the topic is worthy of study, as the school administration has deemed it so. Humanism, ethics, and professionalism are the moral filters of how medical students and residents evolve into physicians (Musick, 1999). Curricula in medical schools need to allow for a thematic longitudinal course that begins in the first year and is sustained through graduation (Lazarus, Chauvin, Rodenhauser, & Whitlock, 2000). This effort would be comprised of an array of pedagogical experiences that would teach theory and knowledge, such as didactic, small group, standardized patients, interdisciplinary conferences, electives, clinical rounds and case conferences (ACGME, 1999).

With most attention in the pre-clinical years being focused coursework on knowledge and analysis, the clinical years of medical school would continue both elements and add components of evaluation of behavior. Case analysis and case discussion would be a prime means of clinical education in medical school (Huijer, van Leeuwen, Boenink, & Kimsma, 2000). Residency education would mirror these efforts as well with an emphasis on practical use of knowledge using case-based examples from inpatient and outpatient experiences, integrating these with new knowledge and analytic skills. As curricula are integrated across the time of residency, case conferences and ethics floor rounds may be the most efficacious way to teach new topics on professionalism and ethics due to the time demands placed on residents.

Assessing Professional Behavior

Assessment in the preclinical setting would consist of small group participation and oral evaluation, written examinations, and standardized patient evaluations. Perhaps the most critical evidence of the attainment of professionalism, however, is behavior of each learner supporting its being put into practice (Shrank, Reed, & Jernstedt, 2004). Codes are of limited value if they are hypothetical. Skills of communication and sound ethical conduct require observational evaluation. In preclinical circumstances, this translates in student-student and student-professional interactions. Adherence to sound academic conduct (e.g. to a school's honor code) is partial evidence to this end. Also, interactions with others in a humane and ethical fashion are of relevance even when cheating and stealing is not involved. Hence, peer and 360° evaluations are essential in professionalism in preclinical education.

In the clinical years and residency, peer and professional evaluation are supplemented by important additional sources. Patients serve as valuable assessors of how professional students behave in their interactions. Standardized patients and other health care staff likewise are valuable to this effort. By the time one has completed medical school and residency, multiple assessments of the humanistic, ethical, and professional facets of student behavior should be evaluated, and if found wanting, remedied. Clinical evaluations would be based on Objective Structured Clinical Examinations (OSCEs), chart reviews, observed or recorded clinical interactions, as well as clinically observed behavior via 360° evaluations by residents, peers, medical personnel, and patients (Singer, 2003). In residency, observation techniques discussed above would be critical in measuring satisfactory professional progress.

CHALLENGES TO THE CODE

As is often the case, this expanded curricular mandate is not funded. No new monies have been allocated for the effort. The hope that future malpractice costs will diminish as a result of these efforts will be of little consolation to medical schools and residency programs. On the other hand, there is a considerable "stick" to reckon with if curricula do not change and if resources are not realigned. Medical schools with meager professionalism efforts can endanger their accreditation, and residencies could not only lose accreditation, but also millions of dollars of Medicare funds. Resources will therefore need to be found or redeployed to allow for both teaching (didactic and analytic) as well as observation.

Resource sharing among medical schools and residency programs may be a prudent economic response. Collaboration with other hospitals, graduate programs in humanities, and with other educational schools may allow for a means to bridge the "professionalism pedagogy gap" that the new accreditation standards have now created. Retraining current faculty through intensive seminars and courses, as well as through sponsorship of graduate degrees in medical ethics and humanities (both masters and doctorate level), would be facilitated by institutional tuition remission and release time.

While some medical schools and residency programs may resist the spending of economic and political capital to put professionalism into practice, they will likely have no choice. Accreditation is the lifeblood to medical education. Foregoing accreditation is the educational funding "third rail." For example, some residency programs recently found out the hard way that by not adhering to ACGME work hour rules, each would be met with loss of accreditation. Professionalism will likely be the next test of medical school and residency program adequacy.

CONCLUSION

The proposed Educational Code of Professionalism is to serve as a means to have the physician-in-training and his or her teacher profess what they strive to be: professionals. It also serves notice that society, physicians, patients, and accreditation bodies hold this commitment with grave seriousness. When all training programs concur that we must teach our students to become professionals, and put resources in place to make this happen, our students and residents can then not only profess their intentions, but also allow them to actualize these ideals in their clinical practice.

REFERENCES

Accreditation Council for Graduate Medical Education (2001). *Outcome project*. Retrieved May 31, 2005, from the Accreditation Council of Graduate Medical Education Website: http://www.acgme.org/outcome/comp/compFull.asp

American Society for Bioethics and Humanities. (2005). The model curriculum project on bioethics and humanities. Retrieved July 6, 2005, from the ASBH website: http://www.asbh.org

Cassel, C. (2002). *Patient safety, professionalism and continuous professional development*. Retrieved May 31, 2005, from the Accreditation Council for Graduate Medical Education website: http://www.acgme.org/outcome/PowerPoint/Cassel.ppt

Cohn, F. & Lie, D. (2002). Mediating the gap between the white coat ceremony and the ethics and professionalism curriculum. *Academic Medicine, 77*, 1168.

Coulehan, J., & Williams, P.C. (2003). Conflicting professional values in medical education. *Cambridge Quarterly of Healthcare Ethics, 12*, 7-20.

Council on Ethical and Judicial Affairs. (2001). *Principles of medical ethics*. Chicago: American Medical Association.

Doukas, D.J. (1991). Autonomy and beneficence in the family: Describing the family covenant. *Journal of Clinical Ethics, 2*, 145-148.

Doukas, D.J. (2003). Where is the virtue in professionalism? *Cambridge Quarterly of Healthcare Ethics, 12*, 147-154.

Fresa-Dillon, K.L., Cuzzolino, R.G., & Veit, K.J. (2004). Professionalism: Orientation exercises for incoming osteopathic medical students and developing class vision statements. *Journal of the American Osteopathic Association, 104*, 251-259.

Jonsen, A.R. (1999). *A short history of medical ethics*. New York: Oxford University Press.

Hatem, C.J. (2003). Teaching approaches that reflect and promote professionalism. *Academic Medicine, 78*, 709-13.

Huijer, M., van Leeuwen, E., Boenink, A., & Kimsma, G. (2000). Medical students' cases as an empirical basis for teaching clinical ethics. *Academic Medicine, 75*, 834-8399.

Kenny, N.P., Mann, K.V., & MacLeod H. (2003). Role modeling in physicians' professional formation: Reconsidering an essential but untapped educational strategy. *Academic Medicine, 78*, 1203-1210.

Kohn, L.T, Corrigan, J.M., & Donaldson M.S. (Eds.). (1999). *To err is human: Building a safer health system*. Washington, DC: National Academy Press.

Lazarus, C.J., Chauvin S.W., Rodenhauser P., & Whitlock R. (2000). The program for professional values and ethics in medical education. *Teaching & Learning in Medicine, 12*, 208-11.

Lehmann, L.S., Kasoff, W.S., Koch, P., & Federman, D.D. (2004). A survey of medical ethics education at U.S. and Canadian medical schools. *Academic Medicine, 79*, 682-9.

Liaison Committee on Medical Education (2005). *LCME accreditation standards*. Retrieved May 31, 2005, from the Liaison Committee on Medical Education website: http://www.lcme.org/standard.htm

Medical Professionalism Project Members: ABIM Foundation, ACP-ASIM Foundation, and European Federation of Internal Medicine. (2002). Medical professionalism in the new millennium: A physician charter. *Annals of Internal Medicine, 136*, 243–246.

Murden, R.A., Way, D.P., Hudson, A., & Westman, J.A. (2004). Professionalism deficiencies in a first-quarter doctor-patient relationship course predict poor clinical performance in medical school. *Academic Medicine. 79*, S46-8.

Musick, D.W. (1999). Teaching medical ethics: A review of the literature from North American medical schools with emphasis on education. *Medicine, Health Care & Philosophy, 2*, 239-54.

Ozar, D. (1995). Profession and professional ethics. In W.T. Reich (Ed.), *Encyclopedia of bioethics* (3rd ed., pp. 2103-2112). New York: Simon & Schuster.

Patenaude, J., Niyonsenga, T., & Fafard, D. (2003). Changes in students' moral development during medical school: A cohort study. *Canadian Medical Association Journal, 168*, 840-844.

Pellegrino, E.D. & Thomasma D.C. (1988). *For the patient's good: The restoration of beneficence in health care.* Oxford, United Kingdom: Oxford University Press.

Pellegrino, E.D. & Thomasma D.C. (1993). *The virtues in medical practice.* Oxford, United Kingdom: Oxford University Press.

Shrank, W.H., Reed V.A., & Jernstedt G.C. (2004). Fostering professionalism in medical education: A call for improved assessment and meaningful incentives. *Journal of General Internal Medicine, 19*, 887-892.

Singer, P.A. (2003). Strengthening the role of ethics in medical education. *Canadian Medical Association Journal, 168*, 854-855.

Surdyk, P.M. (2003). Educating for professionalism: What counts? Who's counting? *Cambridge Quarterly of Healthcare Ethics, 12*, 155-60.

Part Two

TEACHING PROFESSIONALISM

Chapter 4

MEDICAL PROFESSIONALISM
The nature of story and the story of nature

Daniel George, Iahn Gonsenhauser, and Peter Whitehouse
Case Western Reserve University

   All human communities rely on healers to elaborate conceptions of health and wholeness, and apply their expertise for the benefit of individuals and societies. The process of "professionalizing" young doctors in medical schools allows society to train experts who are entrusted with developing the systems of knowledge, the institutions, and the relationships necessary to maintain and improve the health of human individuals and the community at large (Greaves, 2004, p. 67-69). Medical education in the United States has fallen under especially intense scrutiny in recent years for neglecting to explore, adapt, or contemporize the social contract that has long linked healers to their communities, and for failing to curtail the pessimism that runs rampant amongst medical students, diminishing their confidence and making them doubt their abilities to become professionals (Wagoner, 2000). Medical education has even been accused of destroying idealism and creating cynicism in its stead.

   As many have pointed out, the professionalism discourse currently conceived in our medical schools often seems more of a humanizing veneer of platitudes and abstract definitions than an operational ethos in students' lives. Too often, as students wend their way through medical school, a tacit professional socialization occurs, transferring sets of values, beliefs, and behaviors that may be altogether inconsistent with the avowed tenets of medical professionalism (Coulehan, 2000). Noble abstractions are uttered, commendable pronouncements are made, but because there is no sustained attempt to filter them through the cultural realities students face, they are not reinforced and are instead perceived as ivory-tower propaganda.

In this chapter, we consider aspects of medical professionalism that deserve greater conceptual and practical emphasis in medical education and suggest how such ideas and behaviors may be integrated into a medical student's code of ethical responsibility. First we briefly adumbrate the philosophical framework for a curricular reform that reunites the disciplines of public health and medicine into a single complementary program of study that will recapture the balance of knowledge, values, and action that characterizes any healthy polity. Following this conceptual overview, we offer a brief summary of a highly effective elective course called "The Healer's Art," developed by Dr. Rachel Naomi Remen at the University of California at San Francisco (UCSF) School of Medicine and successfully replicated in over 25 medical schools nationwide. "The Healer's Art" is an innovative course predicated on the time-honored art of storytelling, which addresses the growing loss of meaning and commitment experienced by physicians who function under the stresses of the modern health care system (Remen, 2002). Because we find Remen's pedagogical approach in her micro-based course that is concerned with the patient-physician relationship to be exemplary, we will make an argument for employing her techniques at the macro-level of public health matters that concern communities. Next, we will present the plan for a radical curricular reform that is currently being undertaken at our own School of Medicine at Case Western Reserve University (CWRU) in Cleveland, Ohio. Finally, we will provide a detailed sketch of a course called "The World of the Healer" that we propose to offer to fourth-year medical students at CWRU. Our course incorporates many of the same pedagogical principles used by Dr. Remen, particularly the notion that in human communities the most substantive learning takes place through the sharing of stories, and has the similar aim of broadening the horizons of our medical students as they begin to envision their future roles in health organizations. Later, as an appendix, we present the course syllabus in its entirety with the hope that it will lend insight into the creative approaches our institution is taking to nurture the professional growth of our students.

WHAT IS PROFESSIONALISM?

In the debate about professionalism (or any other "ism" for that matter), there is an important semantic point that must be addressed. By its definition, an "ism" is a "suffix denoting action or process" (Webster's, 1961, p. 1198); it is an abstract concept that comes into being only because habitual actions taken by human beings have demanded its reification. "Terrorism," then, refers to the collective actions that have been and may be taken by terrorists, while "patriotism" represents the collective actions taken by a nation's individuals in celebration of a shared culture, and so on. Seen in this light, "medical professionalism"—an admittedly elusive term—must be regarded as an abstraction that owes its existence to the sum of collective professional actions taken by practitioners of the medical trade. Thus, when we talk about "medical professionalism," we are not talking about an abstract, divine ethical code that exists beyond medical students in some far-off Hippocratic empyrean. Rather, we are talking about the sum of virtuous professional actions, past, present, and on into the future, for which professionalism serves as a semantic proxy. Professionalism, then, is something that cannot be embraced through the recitation or memorization of a creed. It is not something that can be duplicated, mass-produced, imprinted, or assigned. It is, rather, a social process that human individuals must achieve through personal apprehension, thoughtful reflection, and most importantly, mindful action. Our medical schools must facilitate the professionalization process by providing a space in which a professional ethos can be adopted, internalized, and transformed by each student. In addition to asking of medical students, "What are your values?," we should also be asking them, "Are you prepared to live for your values?"

There has been a concerted effort to move beyond the inert rhetoric of professionalism by establishing new pedagogical methods to help young medical students articulate the goals and values of their profession, bind these conceptual values to the practical structures they face in the world, and so embody them in their professional careers. But in order to truly foster the essential elements of professionalism that we talk about—altruism, accountability, excellence, duty to service, integrity, respect, empathy, compassion, lifelong learning, and the like—the fledgling healers of our society must see themselves as situated in a particular milieu rife with social, ethical, economic, and environmental exigencies that will influence and shape every interaction they have and every decision they must make as professionals in the field of medicine. Professionalism must become less a patina of well-meaning abstractions and more a deliberate method by which medical education helps its young practitioners attain a more holistic understanding of what it is to be a medical professional practicing in a particular social and historical context.

In the past, professionalism has emphasized the relationships between individual patients and physicians, and not the responsibilities of medicine to society at large. Now, however, a subtle but important shift in focus must occur from private to public. That is, we need a transformative process that takes into consideration the politics of health care, the commercial industry's influence over the direction of medical research and practice, and the natural environment's centrality to public health. Each individual practitioner needs to see his or her potential to influence the future direction of medicine and care for patients in the evolving constraints and opportunities of the new century. Increasingly, the private personal health of the persons under the care of a physician will be more affected by the ravages of environmental toxins, infectious agents, and climate change. Every physician will need to know more about conservation, ecological, evolutionary, and complementary and alternative medicine (White House Commission on Complementary and Alternative Medicine Policy, 2002). When we help students to understand themselves and their surroundings more fully as they gauge and assess their ethical responsibilities and professional growth, we give them the vital support they need to become humble yet confident healers who can protect both individuals and communities, advocate for change, and honor the ever-evolving social contract between healers and society.

It may be fairly asked why medicine must renegotiate its social contract in the first place. After all, in some ways, human communities have never been healthier: People live longer and have a higher quality of life than ever before; birth rates are up; infectious disease rates have never fallen so low. Why must we now "take pause," and in doing so disobey the timeless adage, "If it ain't broken, don't fix it"? (Wear & Kuczewski, 2004, pp.1-10). Ostensibly, it is not medicine itself that needs to be "fixed." It is, rather, that the 21st century world where medicine is now situated has a host of external challenges requiring our future medical practitioners to reconstitute their professional bearings and rethink their social contract in lieu of ever-changing circumstances.

Most problematic to the medical professionals of the future is that the practice of medicine has become enslaved by a business model. This problem needs little elaboration: 45 million uninsured Americans speak volumes about the egregious disparities and inequities that plague our country's managed care system (DeNavas et al., 2003). Young doctors must be aware not only of shifting health care economics, managed care ethics, and modern information systems, but also of the foundations of the inequalities that inhere in the health system they themselves are soon to join. These rising professionals will find themselves in the interstice between the culture of commercial business and the culture of clinical medicine. As such, our medical schools must encourage students to confront the ethical, legal, and professional challenges that they will inherit, and facilitate the conditions in which they can gain full purchase of their surroundings, working toward ethical clarity and conviction in a health care system full of racism, classicism, and intrinsic inequality (Hafferty, 2000, pp. 18-19).

Moreover, we live in an age in which pharmaceutical companies have come to dominate the medical arena—perhaps for better and for worse. From the billions of pills we consume each year to the very conceptions we have about our bodies and minds, sickness and health, and standards of normality and abnormality, the pharmaceutical industry is a cultural juggernaut with incalculable influence over sick individuals, not to mention the doctors who must heal them (Brody, 2005, pp. 82-85). Real-world conflicts of interest, co-optation, gift-giving, over-medication, and the pharmaceutical industry's hand in creating new "diagnostic categories" must be interposed with the abstract professional values of medicine for significant professional transformation to take place. Students must be asked to imagine themselves interacting with the policies, structures, institutions, economic interests, and sundry other antagonists that they will inevitably confront and negotiate with in their professional careers. Medical care cannot be treated as a commodity, or as a prime opportunity for pecuniary improvement, and young doctors must learn to assume personal responsibility for their behavior and resist the temptation of letting personal income trump their commitment to patients' well-being. As medicine becomes more inextricably entangled with industry, we must help to provide educational safeguards to protect the public's health (Kassirer, 2005, p. 207).

The social contract linking the 21st century healer to his or her world will also ineluctably include issues of global and environmental health, as well as an apprehension of the changing demographics of our country. An estimated 35 million people—13 percent of the total population of the United States—are now aged 65 and older. According to the U.S. Bureau of the Census, this percentage will accelerate rapidly beginning in 2011, when the first baby boomers reach age 65. In the next decade, as members of the baby-boom generation advance into their 60s, they will constitute the largest elderly population in our country's history. By the year 2030, it is estimated that nearly one-fourth of the nation's population (70 million) will be age 65 or older, with average life expectancy being 77.5 years for men and 82.9 for women (Greenblat, 2004, pp. 92, 93). As patients will be living longer and suffering more and more from the ravages of airborne environmental toxins, contaminated water, and global climate changes, solutions to these problems will be found not just in caring for affected patients on an individual basis, but in addressing and heading-off the economic, social, and ecological injustices that under gird these problems (Whitehouse, 2004, pp. 43-45). Moreover, the very young in our culture are especially vulnerable to these environmental processes and find their health increasingly neglected by an aging society. Intergenerational inequity is a real issue not to be so easily dismissed by gerontologists as a cultural myth.

Historically, medicine's professional emphasis has been placed squarely on the dynamics of the patient-physician relationship. As revealed by recent developments in the field of narrative medicine, young doctors are expected to be perceptive and empathetic—receptive even to the non-verbal cues of their individual patients (Charon, 2001, p. 288). This emphasis is, and will always be important to the practice of humanistic medicine. But in our 21st century world, medical schools must help students extrapolate a concern for the individual patient to the environment in which those patients live. In this way, professional "duty" will not begin and end at the hospital with the treatment of symptoms and effects. Young doctors can be shown a more nuanced world in which symptoms, maladies, and infirmities are linked to broader causes that may be influenced and even preempted through health policy and public advocacy. In a world of intrinsic limits, scarcity, and environmental constraints, doctors must recognize that the healthiest polity will be one in which all people—for many generations—can live with adequate health and quality of life without destroying the ecological basis of our species and the sense of meaningful community that binds us (Jameton & Pierce, 2004, p. 95). From the spread of infectious diseases to the levels of pollutants and contaminants in a community's air and drinking water, 21st century doctors must acquire a professional ethic that is inclusive of their patients and the global and regional eco-systems in which their patients subsist. Quite simply, the social contract between the healer and the patient must be modernized to meet the challenges of the world we live in.

RACHEL REMEN: THE HEALER'S ART

So what does a commitment to improving the professional development of medical students actually look like? And how can we more effectively ennoble students to become activists on behalf of their patients and communities? As educators in the 21st century, we are charged with developing the pedagogical methods that will engage and empower the future healers of our culture. The traditional educational model that posits the medical educator as an elevated figure who presides over his students with authority and austerity, filling them with biomedical knowledge and infusing them with professional values, is outmoded and no longer tenable in our modern medical environments.

Today's medical students learn in an intricate microsystem of faculty, patients, nurses, and other health care providers. And this microsystem sits within a macrosystem of the academic medical center and university administrators whose worlds are shaped by federal legislation, state budgets, insurance companies, and diverse other chaotic forces (Bickel, 2000, p.184). In the midst of this entropic hospital culture, medical educators must ask ourselves, How can we truly help young students develop and maintain a professional covenant that will hold strong even as they are buffeted by the daily stresses and pressures of a medical world that so often produces cynicism, rancor, and inanition? As scientifically-trained educators, we are accustomed to seeking aggressive solutions to the intractable problems we face; but in our haste to "professionalize" medical students, we may find it far more advantageous to subvert the paradigm by taking pause, and listening to what our *students* have to say about professionalism.

Dr. Rachel Naomi Remen of the UCSF School of Medicine has designed a narrative-based curriculum called "The Healer's Art" that uses storytelling both to empower first- and second-year medical students in perceiving the personal meaning in their daily experience of medicine, and to build a community of inquiry between students and their instructors. This 15-hour, quarter-long elective has been taught annually at UCSF since 1993, and has been successfully implemented in close to 30 other medical schools since. Dr. Remen's innovative educational strategy is based on a "discovery model," which encourages the honest and mutually respectful sharing of experiences, beliefs, and personal truths in a "safe" classroom environment that is free of judgment, one where both students and instructors are intellectual and ethical equals (Remen, 2002, pp. 7-8). Each group meets once a week for three hours, with roughly 10% of the course time being used in a didactic manner (faculty members give formal "seed talk" lectures to provoke ideas in their students). The rest of the session is composed of non-formal, "horizontal" methodologies such as reflection on life experience or personal values, guided imagery, poetry writing and journal keeping (Freire, 1990, p. 57). All participants bring their experiences into the classroom setting and form camaraderie as they come to know one another at greater depth, discover shared professional values, and support one another's struggle to be genuine and true to him/herself in the face of a frenetic professional world. "Healer's Art" instructors do not stand elevated at a podium perorating to a roomful of passive listeners; instead, all sit together face-to-face, side-by-side, co-existing on an even playing field where all voices have equal merit. Predictably, evaluations of the course are uniformly outstanding, and faculty members and students alike describe "The Healer's Art" as unique in their professional development (Remen, 2002, pp. 7-8).

Indeed, there is tremendous potential power in narrative exchange. As the Canadian philosopher Charles Taylor argues, "We cannot but strive to give our lives meaning or substance. . . This means that we understand ourselves inescapably in narrative . . . [which] is an organizing principle of our lives" (Taylor, 1985, p. 51). Dr. Remen's innovative course capitalizes on the transformative potential of human storytelling, namely, its capacity to forge meaningful relationships between people and to help human individuals organize or gain clarity on their experiences, beliefs, and personal ethics and values. Indeed, when we talk about "teaching" professionalism to students, what we are really talking about is the method by which students can come to "author" and enact their own professional code. By telling one's stories in full confidence, and measuring one's day-to-day experiences in medicine with the noble ideals intrinsic to the profession, a student can begin to develop a professional identity, one not foisted upon them by their medical superiors, or put to them in the esoteric form of an antediluvian oath, but is, rather, formed through interactive thought processes with others who are currently dealing with, and have long dealt with, the humbling professional challenges they themselves are facing.

The process of storytelling unleashes students to speak candidly about the real ethical/value issues that they face in their everyday lives without being deadened by the imposing pretense of "professionalism." For it is true that while concepts like altruism, accountability, excellence, duty to service, integrity, respect, empathy, and compassion may seem abstract and sometimes hopelessly unattainable to students, the process of allowing students to tell individual stories that interweave these abstruse elements of professionalism into real-life situations can help them see that they are in fact moral agents operating in a socio-political environment where professional values count. Seen in this light, students can sense the importance and indeed, urgency, of cultivating a personal ethic, and becoming moral agents who can sort out the complexities of the world in which they operate. Sharing personal stories ultimately creates powerful group narratives that will resonate and linger with students far greater than even the most eloquent lecture ever could. Moreover, storytelling can pull both students and faculty members together and create a communal bond that can mitigate against the sense of dislocation, pessimism, and competitiveness so often endemic to medical environments.

Courses like "The Healer's Art" represent the kind of pedagogy that medicine must adopt as it moves forward into the 21st century. Thoughtful self-reflection and mindfulness are the antecedents to meaningful action, and by concentrating our efforts on those areas we nurture the professional healers of the 21st century. Next, we provide an overview of how many of these beliefs are being put into curricular practice at CWRU.

HELPING MEDICAL STUDENTS AUTHOR A NEW SOCIAL CONTRACT FOR A NEW CENTURY OF MEDICAL PRACTICE

Like Dr. Remen, we realize that medical educators must do more than "talk the talk" when it comes to rehabilitating medical professionalism. That said, we are well aware of how daunting curricular reform can be. To paraphrase Dr. Ralph Horowitz, Dean of the CWRU School of Medicine, oftentimes medical schools do a lot of reforming, but not a whole lot of changing. However, at this moment in history, as we recognize the urgency of having a health care system that integrates elements of medicine and public health, curricular reform may be a cultural necessity. Medical educators, policymakers, and others are only now coming to realize the deeply rooted alienation between medicine and public health (R. Horowitz, personal communication, January 2005). Regrettably, the two fields have advanced along different evolutionary tracks and are separated in education by different professional philosophies, content, and modes of instruction; in practice by different goals, delivery systems and authority; and in public support by different levels of investment in infrastructure and societal appreciation. At present, medical students who wish to pursue careers in public health can only do so by earning public health degrees either after graduation from medical school, or through a joint MD/MPH program.

Over the last several decades, the public health infrastructure in local and regional communities has atrophied in large part because of the disinterest of physicians in the integrity of community-level health services. However, the exigencies of our 21st century milieu—from emerging microbial diseases and environmental pollution, to the pharmaceutical industry's ubiquitous presence in our lives, managed care, the looming baby boomer "boom," and the specter of public emergencies linked to acts of terror—all underscore the need for medicine to renew its investment in public health education and infrastructure. Even more, these exigencies provide a clear impetus to create a health care system that interweaves medicine and public health into a single, complementary program of study. To meet this objective, CWRU is currently considering whether to rename its medical school as a school of "Medicine and Health" when it implements a radically-reformed curriculum for the entering class in 2006.

CWRU's revamped curriculum reflects a commitment to a philosophy that entwines medicine and public health in an ongoing lattice of integrated education. We will guide our students to a better understanding of the interplay between the biology of disease and the social context of illness;

between the care of the individual patient and the guardianship of the public's health; and between clinical medicine and population medicine. Epidemiology, quantitative methods, disease prevention, quality assessment and improvement, population medicine, social determinants of disease, health promoting and health damaging behaviors will all be inserted seamlessly into courses that provide the core experiences of medical school. Ultimately, the overarching strategy of our approach will be to blend medical and public health content into the mainstream instruction of medical students in such a way that the two focuses are pedagogically conjoined instead of being regarded as antithetical to one another. As a consequence, the physicians who emerge from this program will be dynamic individuals whose leadership and ethical conduct in science, practice, and health care policy will reflect a keen apprehension of the interplay amongst the most salient themes and pressing needs in modern public health and health care.

While the clinical and basic science education of our students will continue to be of seminal importance in our reformed program, CWRU graduates will also be required to demonstrate mastery in four themes that have been endorsed by our faculty: research and scholarship, clinical mastery, professional leadership, and civic professionalism. The School itself will challenge the profession of medicine to re-imagine itself as responsible not just for the care of patients with illnesses and ailments, but also for the prevention and control of diseases in individuals and communities, and ultimately for the health of United States citizens and for the sustained well-being of our broader world community. It will endow students with all the technical and clinical skills they will need while engaging them in an ongoing, transformative dialogue about what professionalism means, what leadership in society means, and what the 21st century social contract ought to be between a healer and his or her community. In sum, our unprecedented experiment is intended not simply to reform medical education, but to shift existing paradigms in order to reinvent the notion of what a medical education can be.

THE BUILDING BLOCKS OF EDUCATIONAL REFORM

Leadership Training

It goes without saying that medical students need to be schooled in the methods of science and gain exposure to more patients as they refine their clinical abilities. But seldom do we talk about medical schools training their charges in leadership or stressing that a commitment to civic activism is tantamount to research and scholarship. The prosaic medical education models may well develop clinicians capable of caring for individuals, but they are woefully ineffective in producing professional leaders who will advocate for the health of individuals and communities. Leadership is an art form that can be learned, and it can be a critical asset for those who wish to be instruments of change in our contemporary society. In our program, these indispensable skills will be cultivated in special courses designed for medical students by the faculty at the internationally-known Weatherhead School of Management on campus. Facilitators will aid students in developing strategies for exercising leadership in 21st century America, and guide students in envisioning ways in which their particular interests and concerns in public health may be influenced through community action and advocacy. We hope to train doctors who will be able to enact what the philosopher Hannah Arendt calls the "vita active" [active life], a life of initiative, advocacy, and community action, in which they are driven by abiding principle, professional integrity, and a zeal for sustaining and improving the quality of life for human individuals.

Leadership, by its very nature, must be undertaken in human communities. In Arendt's words, "Action is never possible in isolation . . . it always establishes relationships and therefore has an inherent tendency to force open all limitations and cut across all boundaries . . . To act, in its most general sense, means to take an initiative, to begin . . . to set something into motion" (Arendt, 1958, pp.175-180). We wish to help young doctors learn to see themselves as uniquely situated in the modern world as professionals embedded in a variegated cultural landscape that will demand adroit communication skills, tolerance, compassion, and adaptive leadership. To this end, we will form a partnership with the College of Arts and Sciences. We expect that exposing our students to a world outside of medical education will enable them to engage the complexity of the world and develop the critical thinking skills possessed by all thoughtful individuals in a democratic society. This, we expect, will foster a more nuanced sense of what civic engagement in public health is and can be, and demonstrate the social grace, communication skills, humility, and intrapersonal finesse one must possess to "put into motion" any change in modern society. Protean physicians who perceive themselves as potential leaders in society recognize the challenges of the modern world and form concrete strategies for acting on their boldest convictions will be best equipped to protect their communities and care for patients with competence, creativity, and compassion. Our program intends to nurture and encourage this growth.

Service Learning

But it is not enough to merely *teach* leadership; students must be given the opportunity to work hands-on in their community. Cleveland, recently declared by the U.S. Census Bureau (2004) to be the poorest large city in the nation, has a panoply of public health needs that include caring for the uninsured, lowering contaminants in the drinking water, and teaching prevention and nutrition in the city's poorest areas. CWRU School of Medicine realizes that it is embedded in an urban community wherein many individuals suffer from extreme privation and health care inequality. As such, we will offer an opportunity for physicians-in-training to become imbued with a commitment to social service by placing them at volunteer sites (such as the nearby Free Clinic of Greater Cleveland) and with health and social-justice-related volunteer projects being undertaken in the greater Cleveland area (such as community efforts against lead poisoning) (Horowitz, personal communication, 2005). That said, we wish not to be the 800-pound "medical-school guerilla" that descends on a volunteer site, squats awkwardly, and then trundles back to the ivory tower. There must be ample time for our students to reflect on their service, discuss and digest their experiences in the field, and ponder the ranging implications of those experiences. Indeed, only through meaningful reflection and the communal sharing of successes, failures, frustrations, value-judgments, and insecurities through storytelling, can young students distill durable lessons from their service, and absorb those lessons into their professional constitutions (Hefferman, 2001, pp. 2-8). We see it as incumbent on us to help students critically confront the ethical, legal, and professional challenges that they will inherit, and facilitate the conditions in which students can, through committed public service, gain full purchase of their surroundings and work towards ethical clarity and conviction in a health care system full of racism, classism, and intrinsic inequality.

Narrative Emphasis

In the reformed curriculum, courses will be suffused with a narrative emphasis. This means that they are predicated on free inquiry and open dialogue, fully embracing the storytelling process as a means of personal and communal edification. A traditional top-down approach to medical school education will lapse into obsolescence in the 21st century. This outmoded approach involves a narrating subject (the teacher) and patient, receptive objects (the students). Here the teacher talks about reality as if it were motionless, static, compartmentalized, and predictable, and she sees it as her obligation to "fill" the students with the contents of her narration (Freire, 1990, p. 57). But, as previously articulated, students situated in a chaotic medical environment may learn more outside the classroom than within it. As such, we as educators must allow students to speak and express themselves through the honest and mutually respectful sharing of experience. It is our charge as educators to help students gain self-clarity and comprehend their surroundings on their own terms, guiding them in actively assessing their professional growth and development, and authoring their own professional code. By telling one's stories in full confidence and measuring one's day-to-day experiences in medicine with the noble ideals intrinsic to the profession, students will develop professional identities.

Consequently, in our program, an education will not be *bestowed* or *imparted* onto passive students. Instead, with an abiding faith in the consciousness and creativity of our physicians-in-training, we will empower students to learn through a narrative-based "discovery method" in which they take a central role in their own exploration of scientific and ethical values. Educators will be guides and instructors who facilitate the uptake of clinical and biological knowledge and foster the development of professionalism by receiving and adding to the stories brought to them by their students. Only through communication can human life hold meaning; and only those who trust and respect one another can truly communicate. And so, in our curriculum we aim to offer dialogic courses predicated on honesty and reciprocity, which will inspire reflection, action, and increased retention of knowledge among our students.

We are currently in the process of developing a narrative-based course called "The World of the Healer." This elective, intended for fourth-year students, closely mirrors Rachel Remen's "The Healer's Art" course in its format, but differs in its pedagogical emphasis. Presenting a brief maquette of the course may be a way for readers to get a sense of the integrated, student-centered educational atmosphere we are seeking to create.

THE WORLD OF THE HEALER

It is undeniable that scientifically-oriented medicine has become the globally-dominant healing tradition, even though many of the world's citizens have limited access to the technologies of so-called Western allopathic medicine. The issues of environmental sustainability and social justice affect the care of individual patients, as well as the viability of our health care organizations, not to mention the future of our cultures at large.

These challenges require us to broaden our traditional educational goals and help students develop the capacity to care for their communities and their planet with as much solicitude as they are taught to have for individual patients.   Understanding the economic forces at work in their field is a critical part of this education, as is an incorporation of the knowledge and wisdom that the humanities have to offer to future medical professionals. Appreciating the importance of the values embedded in our health care organizations alongside our own should be a vital part of any medical student's educational explorations. As such, our elective course is experience-based and conversation-driven, designed to enable the formation of a learning community that will foster inquiry and allow for the mutually-respectful exchange of stories, experiences, beliefs, values, and goals.

The overall objectives of our course are as follows:

1. To elucidate the meaning of professionalism in medicine in the context of environmental health and medical commerce.
2. To understand, through the exchange of personal stories, the role of money in medicine and to discuss how money and "profit-motive" may affect professional values.
3. To explore how business can both damage and improve the environment.
4. To discover how we relate to our natural environmental systems, and to affirm our responsibility for community health as well as the health of our individual patients.
5. To reaffirm our commitment as society's healers and to rediscover the heart and soul of medical service in the context of our health care organizations.

Much like Rachel Remen's course, we seek to establish a "safe" environment in which stories may be shared in confidence with one's colleagues, and received in a spirit of compassion.   Whereas the usual medical training environment is often judgmental, competitive, unforgiving, and performance-driven, and places students in adversarial relationships with one another, our elective will encourage interpersonal connection and create conditions that allow students to establish comfort and camaraderie with one another and with faculty. Even though faculty members will be present, we will emphasize that there are no "experts" in attendance. It is not the wisdom of individuals that we are after; rather, it is the wisdom of the collective life experience of the group, which is harvested through candid dialogue and experiential learning.

Course materials will be included in a supplemental reader, but readings will not be mandatory.   Literary selections describing the power and influences of money and nature on our lives will be included, along with scholarly papers on relevant topics; these will highlight the themes of the discussions undertaken in the course. There will be no testing and no grading. At the conclusion of the course, each student will be asked to conduct a self-assessment and a course evaluation. Students who attend the sessions will receive a passing mark.

At the start of each session, a senior faculty member will deliver a presentation on the day's topic, a conversation starter. This may be of varying length, and may assume different forms. Nevertheless, the intent of each talk will be the same: to plant ideas to stimulate the conversations for the small-group breakout sessions that will follow. Such an initial talk is an opportunity for students to ponder the implications of the perspective they are hearing, and to reflect on their own values and beliefs in the context of the day's theme.

Small groups are the most intimate form of community that is achieved in the course. Nearly half of the classroom time will be spent in small groups. In these groups, students come to know each other at a new depth. Hopefully, they will discover shared and differing values, gain clarity on their own personal and professional goals, and become more confident and comfortable in asserting themselves with their peers. Ideally, each group will have no more than five students and one faculty member. Ground rules (e.g., that nothing will be shared outside of the classroom, that all discussion will be confidential, that no one will be censured for their views, etc.) will be established before the start of each breakout session, and every participant must agree to abide by these rules before the discussion begins. Groups will be assigned at random. One breakout session will focus on an individual writing assignment, rather than small group discussion.

After the breakout sessions, the entire group will reconvene to share what was discussed in the small group sessions. The speaker who delivered the introductory talk will facilitate the group discussion, establishing an open forum for honest dialogue, where all may share their perspectives without fear of recrimination or reproach. It is in this space that the collective wisdom of the group will be synthesized and "brought home" for all in attendance. We include our course outline as an appendix at the end of the chapter to give a window of insight into what the complexion of each course session will be.

CONCLUSION

In this chapter, we have considered the aspects of medical professionalism that deserve greater conceptual and practical emphasis in medical school education, and have suggested that a curriculum which integrates medicine and public health, encourages service-learning, and fosters narrative reflection about professional values allows students to form a nuanced sense of ethical responsibility and augments their potential to be advocates for community health. The philosophical under-girding of our curricular reform at Case Western Reserve University is one that will reunite the disciplines of medicine and public health into a single complementary program of study and recapture the balance of knowledge, value, and action that characterize any healthy polity.

Obviously, the challenges that we face at our own institution are great. But we believe that the potential benefits of reform are immeasurable, making the risk well worth taking. CWRU is uniquely positioned to build on its history of innovation in education, and the leadership of President Edward Hundert, M.D., a psychiatrist and former dean of medicine at the University of Rochester, is nourishing our efforts and ensuring that the new School of Medicine and Health will truly be linked to the Greater Cleveland community. At this watershed period in history, we seek to embrace our institution's spirit of innovation and develop an exemplary method by which medical students can acquire the clinical mastery, professional values, leadership skills, narrative competency, and mindfulness of public health matters that will allow them to care for individuals, and the communities and ecosystems in which those individuals live.

Indeed, the zeitgeist of our age seems to be prodding medical educators to be more attentive to the social conscience and ethical development of trainees, as a means of creating skilled humanistic physicians to care for individuals and communities in the 21st century. Our country's medical schools must see it as their highest desideratum to help students explore, adapt, and contemporize the social contract that has long linked healers to their communities. The new social contract we must forge with our communities will lead us away from a narrow focus on biological solutions to our health problems and closer to a new paradigm of health, which is better suited to meet the needs of the 21st century. Our professional goals must no longer be self-serving, concerned with economic advancement and scientific developments, and co-opted by the pharmaceutical industry. We need to ask our medical professionals not if they have recited the Hippocratic oath, but if they are living their values. Commitment will come through the creation of transformative learning experiences and pedagogical changes through personally interacting with faculty and sharing individual stories in communities of healers. One would hope that bioethicists, recognizing their roots in environmental and land ethics, would take some initiative in the professional development of doctors and help forge this nexus between healers and their social and natural communities.

Ultimately, it is our hope that the CWRU School of Medicine and Health can be a bellwether for other medical programs in the nation. Medicine in the 21st century presents daunting challenges to our culture, and we must evolve and adapt our pedagogy to train professionals who will be dynamic enough to care for and protect the health of individuals, communities, and ultimately, the planet.

APPENDIX

THE WORLD OF THE HEALER

SESSION 1: IDEOLOGY AND THE MEDICAL PROFESSION

Conversation Starter:

What is a profession? What values underlie medical professionalism? The concept of a value-laden profession will be introduced. What are the roles, relationships, and responsibilities of people who are given the title "professional" by society? The history of the medical profession will be examined and current stresses faced by physicians as individuals and groups will be considered. The roles of the sciences and of commerce in influencing medicine's value system will be illuminated. The notion of "isms" (i.e., ideologies and underlying belief systems) will be presented with reflection on which "isms" undergird our profession.

Breakout Session:

What are values in medicine? How are values formed? Do we agree with these values?

Group Discussion:

Definitions of professionalism. What values anchor professionalism in medicine?

Literary Readings:

Sexton, A., "Doctors"

Williams, W.C., "Mind and Body"

Brody, H., "The Chief of Medicine"

Academic Readings:

Wear, D., & Bickel, J., *Educating for Professionalism: Creating a Climate of Humanism in Medical Education*

Thompson, A., & Temple, N.J., "Medicine and Medical Research: The Case for Reform"

SESSION 2: COMMERCIALISM AND MEDICINE

Conversation Starter:

How money influences medicine and the pharmaceutical industry's influence on medicine will be used as a case example of the economic forces at work in medicine. Conflict of interest will be defined and elaborated upon through the sharing of personal stories. The differences between for-profit and non-profit organizations will be reviewed.

Breakout Session:

How does money affect health? Share stories of times when finances impacted a health outcome in a profound way

Group Discussion:

Breakout groups present one or more of their stories to the whole class. Themes about the effects of money are raised and discussed at greater length

Academic Readings:

Kass, L., "The New Biology: What Price Relieving Man's Estate?"

Kodish, E., Murray, T., Whitehouse, P., "Conflict of Interest in University-Industry Research: Relationships, Realities, Politics and Values"

Whitehouse, P., "Interesting Conflicts and Conflicting Interests"

Bonaccorso, S., Sturchio, J., "Perspectives from the Pharmaceutical Industry"

SESSION 3: COMMERCIALISM AND NATURE

Conversation Starter:

How can businesses promote health or damage it? The idea of business will be introduced and examples given of its effects on the environment, such as mining and agribusiness. Pollution will be considered, as well as efforts to make money by improving environmental health.

Writing Project:

What stories can you share of business helping or hurting nature?

Group Discussion:

Share writing projects.

Literary Readings:

Sandburg, C., "The People, Yes"

Thoreau, H.D., "Walking"

Academic Readings:

Gunther, M., "Soy Lovers, Tree Huggers and Profits"

Hofrichter, R., "Reclaiming the Environmental Debate: The Politics of Health in a Toxic Culture"

SESSION 4: MEDICINE'S OBLIGATION TO THE ENVIRONMENT

Conversation Starter:

Should medicine place greater value in nature? The attitudes of science towards nature will be presented. The dominance of genetic reductionistic approaches will be reviewed and ecological frameworks for a conservation approach to medicine considered against our current paradigms.

Breakout Session:

What are current values towards nature in medicine?

Group Discussion:

Share breakout discussions

Literary Readings:

Emerson, R.W., "Nature"

Carson, R., "Silent Spring"

Academic Readings:

Weinhold, B., "Conservation Medicine: Combining the Best of All Worlds"

Whitehouse, P., "The Rebirth of Bioethics: Extending the Original Formulations of Van Rensselaer Potter"

Aguirre, A., Ostfeld, R., & Tabor, G., "Conservation Medicine: Ecological Health in Practice"

SESSION 5: PROFESSIONALISM IN ORGANIZATIONS

Conversation Starter:

What roles and responsibilities do physicians have in organizational life and towards communities rather than individual patients? Physicians tend to think of themselves as individual agents attempting to help individual patients. However, physicians are also members of health care organizations that have responsibilities to whole communities of patients. The impact physicians can have on their own organizations (health care systems and professional groups, for example) will be considered. Examples of green clinics and physicians groups that are active in social justice issues will be presented.

Breakout Session:

What would ideal mission statements for medical schools look like?

Group Discussion:

Share mission statements.

Literary readings:

Kidder, T., *Mountains Beyond Mountains*

Academic readings:

Wear, D., & Kuzcewski, M., "The Professionalism Movement: Can We Pause?"

Whitehouse, P., & Fishman J., "Justice and the House of Medicine: The Mortgaging of Ecology and Economics"

Jameton, A., & Pierce, J., *The Ethics of Environmentally Responsible Health Care*

REFERENCES

Aquirre, A.A., Ostfield, R.S., Tabor, G.M., House, C., & Pearl, M. (2002). *Conservation medicine: Ecological health in practice.* Oxford and New York: Oxford University Press.

Arendt, H. (1958*). The human condition.* Chicago and London: The University of Chicago Press.

Bickel, J. (2000). Growing seeds: Growing the physicians we need. In D. Wear & J. Bickel (Eds.), *Educating for professionalism: Creating a culture of humanism in medical education* (p. 184). Iowa City: University of Iowa Press.

Bonnaccorso, S., & Sturchio, J. (2003). Perspectives from the pharmaceutical industry. *BMJ, 327,* 863-864.

Brody, H. (1991). The chief of medicine. In *The healer's power* (pp. 1-11). Yale University Press.

Brody, H. (2005). The company we keep: Why physicians should refuse to see pharmaceutical representatives. *Annals of Family Medicine, 3*(1), 82-85.

Carson, R. (1996). *Silent spring.* Upper Saddle River, NJ: Prentice Hall.

Charon, R. (2001). Narrative medicine: A model for empathy, reflection, profession, and trust. *Journal of the American Medical Association, 286*(1803), 288.

Coulehan, J., & Williams, P. C. (2000). Professional ethics and social activism: Where have we been? In D. Wear & J. Bickel (Eds.), *Educating for professionalism: Creating a culture of humanism in medical education* (pp. 57-61). Iowa City: University of Iowa Press.

DeNavas-Walt, C., Proctor, B. D., & Mills, R. J. (2004). *Incomes, poverty, and health insurance coverage in the United States: 2003.* Washington DC: U.S. Census Bureau. Retrieved May 20, 2005, from the U.S. government website: http://www.census.gov/prod/2004pubs/p60-226.pdf

Emerson, R.W. (2004). Nature. In R.S. Gottlieb (Ed.), *This sacred earth: Religion, nature, environment.* New York: Routledge.

Freire, P. (1990*). Pedagogy of the oppressed.* New York, NY: Continuum Publishing Company.

Greaves, D. (2004). *The healing tradition: Reviving the soul of Western medicine.* Oxford; San Francisco: Radcliffe Publishing.

Greenblatt, C. S. (2004). *Alive with Alzheimer's.* Chicago: University of Chicago Press.

Gunther, M. (2003). Soy lovers, tree huggers and profits. *Fortune, 147*(13), 98-100.

Hafferty, F. W. (2000). Professionalism and hidden curriculum. In D. Wear & J. Bickel (Eds). *Educating for professionalism: Creating a culture of humanism in medical education.* (pp. 11-34). Iowa City: University of Iowa Press.

Heffernan, K. (2001). *Fundamentals of service-learning course construction.* Paper presented at the Campus Compact, Brown University.

Hofrichter, R. (2000). *Reclaiming the environmental debate: The politics of health in a toxic culture.* Cambridge, MA: MIT Press.

Horowitz, R. (2005). Case School of Medicine and Health: A proposal for radical reform of medical education. Cleveland OH: CWRU.

Kass, L (2001). *The new biology: What price relieving man's estate?* New York: Seven Bridges Press.

Kassirer, J. P. (2005). *On the take: How America's complicity with big business can endanger your health.* Oxford: Oxford University Press.

Kidder, T. (2003). *Mountains beyond mountains: The quest of Dr. Paul Farmer, a man who would cure the world.* New York: Random House.

Kodish, E., Murray, T., Whitehouse, P. (1996). Conflict of interest in university-industry research relationships: Realities, politics and values. *Academic Medicine, 71,* 1287-90.

Ludmerer, K. (1999). *Time to heal: American medical education from the turn of the century to the era of managed care.* Oxford: Oxford University Press.

Pierce, J., & Jameton, A. (2004). *The ethics of environmentally responsible health care.* Oxford: Oxford University Press.

Remen, R. N. (2002). *Finding meaning in medicine: A resource guide.* Bolinas, California: The Institute for the Study of Health and Illness at Commonweal.

Sandburg, C. (1936). *The people, yes.* New York: Harcourt, Brace.

Sexton, A. (1999). Doctors. In *The complete poems.* Boston: Houghton Mifflin

Taylor, C. (1985). *Human agency and language.* Cambridge: Cambridge University Press.

Thompson, A., & Temple, N.J. (2001). Medicine and medical research: The case for reform. In A. Thompson & N.J. Temple (Eds.), *Ethics, medical research, and medicine commercialism versus environmentalism and social justice.* Dordrecht; Boston: Kluwer Academic Publishers.

Thoreau, H.D. (1993). Walking. In S.J. Armstrong & R.G. Botzler (Eds.), *Environmental ethics: Divergence and convergence* (pp. 108-117). New York: McGraw-Hill.

U.S. Census Bureau. (2004). *American Community Survey.* Retrieved May 20, 2005, from the U.S. government website:
http://www.census.gov/acs/www/Products/Ranking/2003/R01T160.htm

Wagoner, N. E. (2000). Identity purgatory to professionalism. In D. Wear & J. Bickel (Eds.), *Educating for professionalism: Creating a culture of humanism in medical education* (pp. 120-133). Iowa City: University of Iowa Press.

Wear, D., & Bickel, J. (Eds.). (2001). *Educating for professionalism: Creating and climate of humanism in medical education.* Iowa City: University of Iowa Press.

Wear, D., & Kuczewski, M. G. (2004). The professionalism movement: Can we pause? *The American Journal of Bioethics, 4*(2), 1-10.

Webster's third new international dictionary of the English language. (1961). Springfield, MA: Merriam-Webster Inc.

Weinhold, B. (2003). Conservation medicine: Combining the best of all worlds. *Environmental Health Perspectives, 111*(10), A524-9.

Whitehouse, P.J. (2003). The rebirth of bioethics: Extending the original formulations of Van Rensselaer Potter. *American Journal of Bioethics, 3*(4), 26-31.

Whitehouse, P.J. (1999). Interesting conflicts and conflicting interests. *Journal of the American Geriatric Society, 47*(6), 759-61.

Whitehouse, P.J., & Fishman, J. (2004). Justice and the house of medicine. *American Journal of Bioethics, 4*(2), 43-45.

White House Commission on Complementary and Alternative Medicine Policy. (2002). Ch 4: Education and Training of Health Care Practitioners. Retrieved May 1, 2005 from: http://www.whccamp.hhs.gov/finalreport.html

Williams, W.C. (1996). Mind and body. In *The collected stories of William Carlos Williams* (pp. 38-49). New York: New Directions.

Chapter 5

RESPECT FOR PATIENTS

A case study of the formal and hidden curriculum

Delese Wear
Northeastern Ohio Universities College of Medicine

> *I gain truth when I expand my constricted eye, an eye that has only let in what I have been taught to see. (Pratt, 1984, p. 17)*

The formal and hidden curriculum are terms widely used in academic medicine, particularly as they relate to the professional development of students. Indeed, medical educators owe a great debt to Fred Hafferty (1994, 1998), whose work in this area was a well-known distinction used by curriculum scholars and sociologists for decades before he brought it to academic medicine (see, for example, Jackson, 1968; Apple, 1971). William Pinar, perhaps the most acclaimed curriculum theorist of the past several decades, defines hidden curriculum as the "ideological and subliminal message[s] presented within the overt curriculum, as well as a by-product of what is not offered—the null curriculum" (Pinar, 1995, p. 27; for null curriculum see Eisner, 1979; Flinders, Noddings, & Thornston, 1986). In addition to the hidden curriculum, curriculum scholars outside medicine also use a number of other related terms to designate unwanted or unintended outcomes of educational experiences, including the informal curriculum (Pinar, 1995), the unwritten curriculum (Overly, 1970), the unstudied curriculum (Dreeben, 1976), and the unplanned curriculum (Zais, 1976). However, Hafferty, a medical sociologist, diverges from curriculum theorists' conception of informal curriculum as extracurricular experiences such as clubs and student organizations (Pinar, 1995), calling the informal curriculum "the learning that takes play via unscripted and idiosyncratic interactions between and among individuals" (Hafferty, 2003).

But it was the term hidden curriculum that captured the interest of medical educators who find it useful to explain the unintended (and most often negative) attitudes, values, and behaviors acquired by medical students in spite of a carefully planned, formal curriculum. In fact, the current academic conversation on professional knowledge, attitudes and behaviors often turns away from the formal curriculum as a potential site for the development of professionalism in students. In his report, "A Flag in the Wind: Educating for Professionalism in Medicine," written when he was a scholar-in-residence at the AAMC, Thomas Inui maintains this curriculum divide by arguing that "additional courses" on "medical professionalism" are unlikely to fundamentally alter negative influences on professional development (2003, p. 5). Even Hafferty argues that "you don't fix the 'bad stuff' being wrought in these shadow-curricula by focusing your remedial efforts solely within the formal curricula" (2003). While I agree that our efforts should not be "solely" within the formal curricula, I also believe that that work in that domain offers great possibilities for the development of professional attitudes in students, particularly when focusing on respect for patients, arguably one of the most foundational of all professional attributes.   In this chapter, I challenge the belief that the formal curriculum should be largely passed over in our pursuit of identifying and changing elements in the social life and organizational culture of medical education linked to both desirable and undesirable attitudes, beliefs, and behaviors in medical students. But first we need to become far more critical in our thinking about the formal and hidden curriculum.

In medical education, curriculum work is rarely a critical activity. In fact, it is most often tethered to the nuts-and-bolts objectives-content-instruction-evaluation paradigm, with little inquiry into the possible social effects of the formal curriculum on students. When we wring our hands about unprofessional attitudes among students, particularly disrespectful attitudes toward patients, we rarely look to the formal curriculum as an explicit or implicit source of such attitudes, believing that the culprit is the hidden curriculum, and the hidden curriculum is elsewhere—those nasty hierarchical rituals enacted in surgery witnessed by students, for example, or the messages about equity and justice sent to students as they learn almost exclusively on "house patients."

What happens when we take a critical look at the ways we address respect for patients in the formal curriculum, but this time for its possible unintended outcomes? The word *critical* is key here as we focus on the formal curriculum as a source that promotes both respectful and disrespectful attitudes toward patients, particularly those from nondominant cultural groups. Thus, I first offer a brief outline of what critical curriculum work entails.

CRITICAL CURRICULUM WORK

To do critical curriculum work is to reflect on our own, the dominant culture's, and the medical profession's deepest held beliefs about what is important for doctors to know and how they are to behave, then investigating how these beliefs show up in what and how we teach. Critical curriculum deliberations signal an ongoing search for the influences of power, tradition, and politics on the structure of the curriculum, even current sacrosanct movements surrounding professional development and competencies. Common questions in critical inquiry include: *Who gets to decide what's important to learn, and who does not? How is the curriculum organized? Who benefits from this organization? What domains of knowledge are left out? What are the explicit and implicit messages students receive through their curriculum experiences?* Such inquiry also implies an exploration into cultural assumptions about health and illness that bias what we teach, raising questions about race, class, and gender as they leak (or don't leak) into the formal curriculum (Wear, 2003). Critical curriculum work looks for ways biomedicine configures and "fixes" patients and illness, resulting in little curriculum space for the cultural, social, and historical conditions that influence human experience (Aull & Lewis, 2004). In other words, critical curriculum work offers a way for medical educators to examine the politics of medical education, including "how we make meaning of commonplace events, the purpose and goals of . . . . [medical] education, how [medical] schools are structured . . . the way students are perceived and treated, the curriculum we use" (Leistyna, Woodrum, & Sherblom, 1996, pp. v-vi).

Medical educators who assume a critical stance toward their work take on a role unlike most of their peers. Like Edward Said's description of the intellectual, the critical medical educator's role

> has an edge to it, [that] cannot be played without a sense of being someone whose place it is to raise embarrassing questions, to confront orthodoxy and dogma (rather than produce them), to be someone who cannot easily be co-opted by governments or corporations, and whose raison d'etre is to represent all those people and issues that are routinely forgotten or swept under the rug. (Said, quoted by Aull & Lewis, 2004)

Critical investigations of the curriculum are guided by a belief that both the formal and hidden curricula are in a tangled knot, and how students experience that knot never matches our intentions. With that in mind, here I provide a critical assessment of cultural competency, a curriculum project in U.S. medical education that ostensibly fosters the development of respect, a value repeatedly cited in the professionalism discourse.

CASE STUDY: A CRITICAL APPROACH TO CULTURAL COMPETENCY

Cultural competency is on the front curriculum burner in U.S. academic medicine. It took some time to arrive here; multicultural efforts have been present in other educative settings since the 1960s, the "fallout of a political project to neutralize Black rejection of the assimilationist curriculum models that were in place in the 1960s" (McCarthy, 1990, p. 47). Most of these various approaches—multiculturalism, diversity, cultural competency, and so on—share the same formal curriculum goals of "sensitizing" students from the dominant culture to minority "differences," toward an end of recognizing and responding "appropriately" to cultural features that affect medical care. These attitudes and behaviors are foundational to professionalism, no matter which group is beating the drums (AAMC [1998], ACGME [2000], ABIM [1995], etc.). But I also propose that such efforts have hidden or unintended components that can actually lead to the erosion of professional attitudes toward patients, particularly in the area of respect.

The most consistent critique of cultural competency is that its approaches are rarely concerned with a critique of systems of oppression (Banks & Banks, 2001; Giroux, 2000; Gordon, 2001; Parker & Lynn, 2002; Sleeter, 2001), that its approaches often conflate race and ethnicity (Sleeter, 2001), and that its approaches rarely address social class (Sleeter, 2001). Regarding ethnicity, Sleeter argues that because ethnicity "does not structure the life chances of European Americans after two or three generations," critiques of oppressive cultural structures and practices are rarely built into cultural competency approaches. Racism, on the other hand, is "deeply structured into society, changing its face but not its basic nature over time. . . . [and] is maintained by social institutions" (Sleeter, p. 91). But when cultural competency is framed around "other" cultures, addressing stereotypes without examining the structural inequality found in social institutions, it "gives the illusion of doing something constructive" (Sleeter, 2001, p. 91). "Cultural differences are a part of [cultural competency]," Sleeter continues, "but in the context of the 'savage inequalities' that characterize U.S. society, cannot receive the great bulk of attention" (p. 91). Cornel West (1992) similarly critiques approaches to culture, arguing that serious discussions about race in the U.S. must begin not with the "problems" or particular "issues" of nondominant groups

> but with the flaws of American society—flaws rooted in historical inequalities and longstanding cultural stereotypes. . . . How we set up the terms for discussing racial issues shapes our perception and response to these issues. As long as black people are viewed as "them," the burden falls on blacks to do all the "cultural" and "moral" work necessary for healthy race

relations. The implication is that only certain Americans can define what it means to be American—and the rest must simply "fit in." (p. 24)

In addition, most approaches to cultural competency are truncated because they don't even delve into the origins of difference. Ogbu's (1992) classification of minority groups or minority status into three groups is a critical tool. He suggests that "to understand what it is about minority groups, their cultures and languages that makes . . . learning difficult for some but not for others, we must recognize that there are different types of minority groups or minority status" (p. 8); that is, there are minority groups that are (1) autonomous, (2) immigrant or voluntary, and (3) castelike or involuntary. Autonomous minorities are persons who are minorities in the numerical sense, like Mormons, the Amish, or Jehovah's Witnesses. Immigrant or voluntary minorities include persons who have voluntarily moved to a country or region, usually for better economic opportunities or for more desirable political conditions. Sometimes these groups have trouble because of cultural or language differences. Some "do not experience lingering, disproportionate . . . failure"; others do (Ogbu, p. 8). Castelike or involuntary minorities are those who were originally brought to a country against their will, usually through "slavery, conquest, colonization, or forced labor. . . . Thereafter, these minorities were often relegated to menial positions and denied true assimilation into the mainstream society. . . . It is involuntary minorities that usually experience greater and more persistent difficulties" (p. 8). Like the conflation of race, ethnicity and other "differences," examination of minority groups or minority status along these dimensions is not included in cultural competency efforts, which sends a message to students by omission that a more nuanced consideration of cultural differences is not important.

In fact, most cultural theorists would argue that cultural competency approaches rarely address sticky political issues in U.S. culture, particularly those surrounding race. Patricia Williams suggests that in the U.S.—and very much at play in medicine—race "tends to be treated as though it were an especially delicate category of social infirmity . . . like extreme obesity or disfigurement" and that those who privilege themselves as "un-raced" (usually white people who purport to be "totally objective" and never "see" skin color) are "always anxiously maintaining that it doesn't matter" (1998, pp. 8-9). But in medicine we know that race does matter on multiple levels, a point dramatically made in the disturbing Institute of Medicine study *Unequal Treatment: Confronting Racial and Ethnic Disparities in Health Care* (2002), and in the daily nuances of doctor-patient interactions.

As I have argued elsewhere (Wear, 2003), cultural competency approaches are important, even "well meaning," but are so limited that any one of them used as the sole approach to the complex interplay between medicine and culture can actually do as much harm as good. In addition to steering clear of critiques of oppressive structures and practices, these approaches do not require medical students from dominant racial groups to think, for example, about their African-American patients' experiences of living in a racist culture, or how everyday medical practices themselves can be racist (Calman, 2000). Moreover, cultural competency approaches do not require students to reflect critically on how their own biases and prejudices are likely to leak undetected into their interactions with all patients. These leaks are the "hidden faces" of racism that are not overt individual acts but the "multiple, subtle ways in which it is constantly deployed" (Lopez, 2001, p. 30). Learning to recognize and respond to cultural features that affect clinical care—one common definition of cultural competency, and indeed, professionalism—does not address, much less attempt to erase, the hidden faces of racism, classism, xenophobia, or any other belief systems that can operate concurrently even as students acquire culturally-specific knowledge and skills. Thus, an unintended message students receive from cultural competency approaches that shy away from scrutiny on self and professional practices is that such critical examination is not necessary if one just learns, in a rational way, about "other" cultures. Such knowledge will supposedly override one's biases and prejudices, or at least make them invisible to patients.

And let us not forget that this is the golden age of "competency," which has turned the attempt to understand patients in all their varieties into data sets to be "mastered," i.e. if Native American then this, if Jehovah's Witness then that. Yet such understandings are complex processes, not simplified products of various "trait" lectures on race, ethnicity, religion, social class, or sexual orientation, which ultimately lead to stereotyping, overgeneralizing, essentializing, and viewing differences as deficiencies (Ford, 1999, p. 9). Ford argues that understanding patients' social and cultural environments is not a competency at all but rather "a process of becoming . . . a perspective or a shared frame of reference from which reality is perceived . . . a way of being, perceiving, thinking, and acting in the world in ways that symbolize the equal respect of all humanity" (Ford, 1999, p. 4).

An article in the *Journal of Pediatrics* (Flores, 2000) provides a clear example of the trait approach to cultural competency and the unspoken messages affixed to such an approach. The article focuses on a single group—Latinos—"rather than a cursory survey of the cultures of multiple groups" (p. 14) to show how culture affects clinical care. In spite of several caveats inserted throughout the article, such as "individuals subscribe to group norms to varying degrees," or "a patient's health beliefs and practices arise from a combination of normative cultural values together with personal experience and perceptions" (p. 15), the article focuses on Latino culture in a 5-component cultural competency model that includes not only demographics and language but also the potentially essentializing components of "normative cultural values," "folk illnesses," and "parent/patient beliefs." Without a doubt, the information provided in articles like this offers care givers important information that can directly affect their patients' health; it can also, if not used with critical discernment, lead to an inappropriately normative response to a Latino/a patient. And while the authors caution that a "wealthy Cuban American" may have values different from a "first-generation Mexican American," they still maintain that a cultural competency model is clinically useful regardless of patients' ethnicity. Unfortunately, this article, like most that address cultural competency in medicine, does not address the fact that every person exists at the intersection of race, ethnic or national identity, religion, social class, and sexual identity (among others), yet each person seems to be fair game for cultural competency categorization into any one of these. As Macedo (1996) points out, "to be reductionistic is to simplify a particular phenomenon so as to mask its complexity" (p. 36), which is what happens when cultural competency approaches pull out one dimension of an individual's identity as the source for understanding who they are.

And when "competency" is the goal, students' gazes remain fixed on "others"—often those who are not white, middle class, English speaking, able-bodied, Judeo-Christian—and not on themselves and the structures of their profession as they assume postures of neutrality and objectivity in their dealings with such patients. That is, they position themselves in the viewing box as the "normal" ones. Among many the cultural divides in the U.S. (e.g. rich/poor, heterosexual/homosexual, able-bodied/disabled, doctor/patient), Patricia Williams (1998) suggests that the racial divides are exacerbated by a "welter of little lies":

White people are victims. Poor Bangladeshies are poor because they want to be. Poor white people are poor because rich Indians stole all the jobs under the ruse of affirmative action. There is no racism in the marketplace. . . . Immigrants are taking over the whole world, but race makes no difference. . . . If some people are determined to be homeless, well then let them have it, if being homeless is what they like so much. (p. 10)

When attempting to provide patients with culturally competent care, what do students "do" with these "little lies" circulating around them and their patients? If the formal curriculum doesn't deal with them directly, these cultural beliefs take up residence in the hushed (but oddly informally sanctioned) corridor talk among students and residents, in the shorthand jargon they use to categorize particular kinds of patients, or in their way of making sense of patients unlike themselves.

Like other models often used in medicine (e.g. the biopsychosocial model), cultural competency is grounded in rationality. Indeed, why would the word "competency" be affixed to the word culture if there were not a belief that culture is something to be learned and tested for evidence of its "mastery"? The *OED* defines competence as "sufficiency of qualification; capacity to deal *adequately* with a subject" [italics added]; *Webster's Third International Dictionary* defines it as "the quality or state of being functionally adequate or of having sufficient knowledge, judgment, skill, or strength." As such, competence is a wildly inappropriate choice of words to describe the process of understanding and respecting cultural differences among all of us. In fact, this undertaking involves not only an "adequate" or baseline cognitive or analytic component—understanding the central beliefs, values, practices, and paradoxes of nondominant cultures, but also an emotional component—the "ability to assume genuine interest in, and to maintain respect for, different (especially counterpart) values, traditions, experiences, and challenges" (Koehn & Rosenau, 2002, p. 110).

The latter is *not* a competency. Moreover, assuming interest in and maintaining respect for patients whose cultural beliefs and behaviors are often antithetical to one's own, particularly when one is not interested in or respectful of such beliefs and behaviors, is not addressed in most current cultural competency curricula (or professionalism curricula for that matter). Yet confronting these lapses in respect involves the difficult, lifelong, always unfinished work of unlearning biases and prejudices, which is not amenable to the whole notion of competency. Instead, it is the self-critical, reflective work individuals must engage in repeatedly, honestly, and concurrently with the cognitive component of cultural competency, or else "understanding" is reduced to "simplifying."

Stepping back, then, to view cultural competency critically in terms of the formal and hidden curriculum, we might make the following observations: The formal curriculum of cultural competency efforts instructs students that differences among patients based on gender, race, ethnicity, national origins, social class, physical or intellectual abilities, sexual identity, or religious beliefs can be and must be known, understood, and respected to maximize their efforts at restoring and maintaining health. The hidden curriculum of these same efforts—what we don't want students to take away from these experiences, but they do, anyway—is that (1) doctors can "achieve" cultural competency by learning sets of other-directed knowledge and behaviors without addressing the all-too-real effects of their biases and prejudices on persons from non-dominant cultures who live in a white-dominated, heterosexist, religiously intolerant, and rabidly nationalistic culture; and (2) doctors can "achieve" cultural competency (and be assessed, for example, through standardized patients) without recognizing and critically addressing structural inequalities in medicine and the social sources of suffering.

WHERE TO NEXT? A PEDAGOGY OF DISCOMFORT

In spite of its potentially negative hidden messages, cultural competency approaches, along with other efforts under the more general rubric of professional development, can be significant, meaningful attempts of medical educators to move medical students toward greater respect for patients in all their variabilities. But as I have attempted to show in a critical reading of this approach, cultural competency approaches have hidden messages that, when read by medical students in the midst of their intense socialization into the profession, may lead them to a view of patients that is superficial, unreflective, even disrespectful, even though they can "perform" otherwise under the scrutiny of a rater. When designated as a competency, culture comes to be viewed as content to be mastered, something on which one can be tested. Given the limitations and possible unintended outcomes of such cultural competency approaches, then, I propose that cultural competency be folded into a pedagogy of discomfort, which may move students to a greater respect and empathy for patients across cultural variables.

Megan Boler, who developed the idea of a pedagogy of discomfort, urges educators of all stripes "to engage in critical inquiry regarding values and cherished beliefs, and to examine . . . how one has learned to perceive others" (1999, p. 176). If we look beyond the simplified data "unearthed" about patients by use of various cultural competency approaches, we find vast worlds of unspoken, unacknowledged "values and cherished beliefs" students use in their history taking and questioning strategies, many of them taught or reinforced by their medical education, some of them reinforced by cultural competency approaches.

But critical reflection on one's values and beliefs (and how one has learned them) is only the first step in a pedagogy of discomfort. The critical inquiry Boler describes moves beyond critical reflection, for stopping there runs the risk of reducing the complexities and contradictions of the social world into an "overly tidy package that ignores our mutual responsibility to one another" (p. 177). Stopping there, she also argues, may evoke some honest self-assessment of biases but nothing more, with no significant changes to oneself or the way one views or treats others. A pedagogy of discomfort thus moves critical reflection into the realm of culture, where we examine how the dominant culture shapes the ways we see the world—a stark contrast to the trait-seeking, test-for-mastery impulse of cultural competency where no such questions are posed. For medical students, this involves scrutinizing not only the dominant U.S. culture but also the formidable medical culture that tells and shows them, via a competency orientation, how health, illness, and caregiving relate to persons from nondominant cultures. In fact, interesting questions can be raised "about an institution primarily composed of members of the dominant class ... to interpret and read signs of illness and health in nondominant persons, not to mention non-dominant persons' relationships to their communities" (Stanford, 2003, p. 34). Moreover, when an examination of culture is focused on learning about the health beliefs of various "other" groups and not on ways one's thinking is shaped, what students learn are "inscribed habits of (in)attention" built on social and economic hierarchies (Boler, p. 180).

If medical educators were to use a pedagogy of discomfort alongside a cultural competency approach or within various professionalism curricula, students would be urged to recognize the selectivity of what they see and to whom/what they give attention. They would examine how this selectivity has evolved in all of us, learned through families, educational experiences, religion, and medical training, all which have very particular incentives and disincentives to construct the world in particular ways. For example, medical students—most of them coming from middle range or economically privileged classes (AAMC, 2001)—would begin to recognize, undoubtedly with some discomfort, that they have great incentives to remain privileged, that their world view is based on their social status and medical training, and that the way they explain poverty, for example, is based on selective sight arising from social status. Similarly, medical educators engaged in a pedagogy of discomfort would come to recognize how the curriculum they construct focuses on a doctor-patient relationship that keeps the doctor firmly in charge how that relationship is constructed, and the incentives they have to keep the relationship functioning that way. This, I argue, informs cultural competency approaches, and in a larger sense, goes to the heart of professionalism in medicine.

Laurie Abraham's celebrated *Mama Might Be Better off Dead: The Failure of Health Care in Urban America* (1994) provides a stinging example of selective sight. Abraham tells the story of one woman who suffered from a severe case of hives that was caused by her allergies to cats, yet she repeatedly refused to get rid of them. Her doctor was angry at her for what appeared to be a simple solution to the problem; only later did he learn that if she got rid of the cat, she believed there was nothing to protect her kids against rats (1994, p. 127). This doctor may have taken a "good" history, but this horrific dimension of her life had remained unknown to him, even though he may or may not have been schooled in cultural competency. It remained unknown to him because of selective sight, which arises from not only his social status but from the hidden ideological and subliminal messages presented to him throughout his medical training within the formal curricula, and as by-product of what is rarely offered to trainees and practicing physicians: a critique of social oppression in all its varieties, how the culture of medicine responds to such oppression, or how individual doctors respond to patients' suffering brought about by social oppression. Moreover, Boler argues that "what is at stake is not only the ability to empathize with the very distant other, but to recognize oneself as implicated in the social forces that create the climate of obstacles the other must confront" (p. 166). This is key: weaving a pedagogy of discomfort into cultural competency approaches requires students to look at their own complicity in creating "climates of obstacles," no matter how subtle.

Like many scholars (Booth, 1988; Brooks, 1992; Nussbaum, 1990) over the past several decades, Boler cites engagement with literature as one vehicle for a pedagogy of discomfort to do its work, one way to develop more respect and empathy for "the very distant other." But she warns that "mere" reading is not necessarily linked to recognizing social practices that harm patients' health, any more than "mere" competency approaches to culture. Instead, Boler argues that "at minimum an active reading practice involves challenging . . . assumptions and world views" (p. 166). That is, to refuse to engage in the world outside a text and to deny any complicity with the social conditions illuminated by that text suggests a passive reading practice that does not translate to anything beyond the actual reading. For example, readers may be outraged by the domestic violence portrayed in Anna Quindlen's *Black and Blue* (1998), the vitriolic racism and incest revealed in Ruthie Bolton's *Gal* (1994), the poverty-level wages and work conditions described by Barbara Ehrenreich in *Nickel and Dimed: On (Not) Getting By in America* (2002), but if the outrage stops there, the respect and empathy readers have for those characters may not extend to others in similar circumstances in the "real" world—to patients, for example, and the worlds they inhabit.

What we need in our classrooms is discomfort, yes, but discomfort that keeps actively moving or else the texts (novels, nonfiction, case studies, panels of patients or other testimonies, or any similar genres) turn into "objects of easy consumption" (Boler, p. 169), just like the "competencies" attached to culture. Boler wants students (and those of us who teach them) not to be spectators of different "others," live or fictional, but rather to be *witnesses*. Witnessing, Boler writes, is a "process in which we do not have the luxury of seeing a static truth or fixed certainty" (p. 186), which is suggested at least implicitly by various approaches to cultural competency that focus on group values, beliefs, or behaviors.   Rather, witnessing is a "dynamic process," an "invitation to question," a willingness to examine our "historical responsibilities and co-implication" in the difficulties faced by groups of people set apart from the dominant culture (p. 186). Thus, if we want students to become more than learned spectators, if we want them to become witnesses, we must urge ways of reading that move them to recognize their impulse to judge others, fictional and "real."   Boler argues that such readings show us people and situations that exceed our frame of reference:

> [R]ecognizing my position as "judge" granted through the reading privilege,
> I must learn to question . . . any particular response: My scorn, my evaluation
> of others' behavior as good or bad, my irritation—each provides a site for
> interrogation of how the text challenges my investments in familiar cultural
> [including medicine's] values . . . I can identify the taken-for-granted social
> values and structures of my own historical moment which mirror those
> encountered by the protagonist. (p. 170)

Barbara Ehrenreich's *Nickel and Dimed* (2001), a first-hand account of how millions of American work full-time for poverty-level wages, provides a compelling possibility for the kind of witnessing Boler describes. Ehrenreich, a Ph.D. in biology and prolific author, moves to three locations and accepts work as a waitress, hotel maid, house cleaner, nursing home aide, and Wal-Mart salesperson, never disclosing her "real" life. She commits to living on the wages offered by whatever job she takes, and quickly realizes that one job is usually not enough. She learns not only how difficult it is to find decent housing and reliable transportation, but how important it is not to get sick because of lost wages. And she also learns how one's spirit can be eroded day after day, how conceptions of work can be worlds apart depending on what one does. She learns a "great truth" about low-wage jobs—that often "nothing happens, or rather the same thing always happens, which amounts, day after day, to nothing" (p. 186). She writes about her job at Wal-Mart:

> You could get old pretty fast here. In fact, time does funny things when there
> are no little surprises to mark it off into memorable chunks, and I sense that
> I'm already several years older than I was when I started. In the one full-
> length mirror in ladies' wear, a medium-tall figure is hunched over a cart, her
> face pinched in absurd concentration—surely not me. How long before I'm
> as gray as Ellie, as cranky as Rhoda, as shriveled as Isabelle? . . . What you
> don't necessarily realize when you start selling your time by the hour is that
> what you're actually selling is your life. (p. 187)

Now, it is possible, even likely, for students to feel empathy for Ehrenreich and the women's lives she so vividly describes, but it is also possible that such empathy decontextualizes the very social problems facing these and the millions of other women just like them. Medical educators who choose a pedagogy of discomfort alongside a cultural competency approach could use Ehrenreich's text to challenge rigid patterns of thinking about those who are economically disadvantaged, urging readers beyond empathic identification with the lives Ehrenreich describes to the very culture in which they will practice. As witnesses (versus mere spectators), students would learn to engage in individual and collective self-reflection, "to develop accountability for how we see ourselves . . . [to] question cherished beliefs" (Boler, p. 188). As witnesses, students may find themselves at a juncture where they must decide how they will enact commitments newly gleaned from identification with texts: Some may intervene in conversations where disrespect for patients is part of the normal conversation; others may take risks expressing alternative perspectives on race or sexual identity; still others may choose career paths of action "as a result of learning to see differently" (p. 199).

CONCLUSIONS

A pedagogy of discomfort, which works toward developing deeper respect for others as it challenges our world views, is one way to make more visible some of the hidden aspects of the medical curriculum. Here I suggest that the reading of literary texts, used in a spirit of discomfort, might make visible some of the unintended messages of cultural competency approaches that lead only to "spectating" others. When medical educators adopt a critical stance toward the medical curriculum, openings for a pedagogy of discomfort become all too apparent in any course on the doctor-patient relationship, in any clinical rotation, in any classes focusing on professionalism, bioethics, humanities, or culture. Moreover, a pedagogy of discomfort that relies on "stories, parables, chronicles, and narratives" is a compelling way to trouble mindsets imposed by thinking schematically about human differences: doctors like us are here, patients like them are over there. These mindsets, our rarely examined mindsets, are "like eyeglasses we have worn a long time. They are nearly invisible; we use them to scan and interpret the world and only rarely examine them for themselves" (Delgado, 2000, p. 61). These, too, are the eyeglasses of cultural competency and professionalism that have been uncritically accepted by the academic medicine community. It's time to wipe off, or take off, the glasses.

REFERENCES

American Association of Medical Colleges. (1998). *Medical school objective project.* Retrieved February 4, 2004 from the AAMC website: http://www.aamc.org/meded/msop/start.htm

American Association of Medical Colleges. (2001). Parents' education and income level of all medical matriculates: 2000. Washington, DC: AAMC.

American Board of Internal Medicine. (1995). *Project* professionalism. Retrieved January 15, 2004 from the ABIM website: http://abim.org/pubs/profess.pdf

Abraham, L.K. (1994). *Mama might be better off dead: The failure of health care in urban America.* Chicago: University of Chicago Press.

Accreditation Council for Graduate Medical Education. (2000). *Outcome project.* Retrieved January 15, 2004 from the ACGME website: http://www.acgme.org/outcome/comp/compfull.asp

Apple, M. (1971). The hidden curriculum and the nature of conflict. *Interchange, 2*(4), 27-40.

Aull, F., & Lewis, B. (2004). Medical intellectuals: Resisting medical orientalism. *Journal of Medical Humanities, 25, 87-108.*

Banks, J.A., & McGee Banks, C.A. (2001). *Handbook of research on multicultural education.* San Francisco: Jossey-Bass.

Boler, M. (1999). *Feeling power: Emotions and education.* New York: Routledge.

Bolton, R. (1994). *Gal.* New York: Harcourt Brace.

Booth, W. (1988). *The company we keep: An ethics of fiction.* Berkeley: University of California Press.

Brooks, P. (1992*). Reading for the plot: Design and intention in narrative.* Cambridge: Harvard University Press.

Calman, N. (2000). Out of the shadows. *Health Affairs, 19,* 170-174.

Delgado, R. (2000). Storytelling for oppositionists and others: A plea for narrative. In R. Delgado & J. Stefancic (Eds.), *Critical race theory* (pp. 60-70). New York: NYU Press.

Dreeben, R. (1976). The unwritten curriculum and its relation to values. *Journal of Curriculum Studies, 8*(2), 111-124.

Ehrenreich, B. (2001). *Nickel and dimed: On (not) getting by in America.* New York: Henry Holt.

Eisner, E. (1979). *The educational imagination.* New York: Macmillan.

Flinders, D., Noddings, N., & Thorston, S. (1986). The null curriculum: Its theoretical basis and practical implications. *Curriculum Inquiry, 16*(1), 33-42.

Flores, G. (2000). Culture and the patient-physician relationship. *Journal of Pediatrics, 136,* 14-23.

Ford, T. (1999). *Becoming multicultural: Personal and social construction through critical teaching.* New York: Falmer Press.

Giroux, H. (2000). Insurgent multiculturalism and the promise of pedagogy. In E.M. Duarte & S. Smith (Eds.), *Foundational perspectives in multicultural education* (pp. 195-212). New York: Longman.

Gordon, B. (2001). Knowledge construction, competing critical theories, and education. In J.A. Banks & C.A. McGee Banks (Eds.), *Handbook of research on multicultural education* (pp. 184-199). San Francisco: Jossey-Bass.

Hafferty, F.W., & Franks, R. (1994). The hidden curriculum, ethics teaching, and the structure of medical education. *AcademicMedicine, 69,* 861-871.

Hafferty, F.W. (2003, November). The hidden curriculum and medical education. Paper presented at the annual meeting of the American Association of Medical Colleges, Washington, DC.

Koehn, P.H., & Rosenau, J. N. (2002). Transnational competence in an emergent epoch. *International Studies Perspectives, 3, 105-127.*

Institute of Medicine. (2002). *Unequal treatment: Confronting racial and ethnic disparities in health care.* Retrieved July 1, 2005, from http://www.iom.edu/report.asp?id=4475

Inui, T. (2003). *A flag in the wind: Educating for professionalism in medicine.* Washington, DC: AAMC.

Jackson, P. (1968). *Life in classrooms.* New York: Holt, Rinehart, & Winston.

Leistyna, P., Woodrum, A., & Sherbloom, S.A. (Eds.). (1996). *Breaking free: The transformative power of critical pedagogy.* Cambridge, MA: Harvard Educational Review Reprint Series 27.

Macedo, D.P. (1996). Literacy for stupidification: The pedagogy of big lies. In P. Leistyna & S.A. Sherblom (Eds.), *Breaking free: The transformative power of critical pedagogy* (pp. 31- 57). Cambridge, MA: Harvard University Press.

McCarthy, C. (1990). Race and education in the United States: The multicultural solution. *Interchange, 21*(3), 45-55.

Nussbaum, M. (1990). *Love's knowledge.* New York: Oxford University Press.

Lopez, G.R. (2001). Re-visiting white racism in educational research: Critical race theory and the problem of method. *Educational Researcher, 30*(1), 30.

Ogbu, J.U. (1992). Understanding cultural diversity. *Educational Researcher, 21*, 5-14.

Overly, N. (1970). *The unstudied curriculum.* Washington, DC: Association for Supervision and Curriculum Development, Elementary Education Council.

Parker, L., & Lynn, M. (2001). What's race got to do with it? *Qualitative Inquiry, 8*(1), 7-22.

Pinar, W.F. (Ed.). (1995). *Understanding curriculum.* New York: Peter Lang.

Pratt, M.B. (1984). Identity: Skin/blood/heart. In E. Bulkin, M.B. Pratt, & B. Smith (Eds.), *Yours in struggle.* New York: Long Haul Press.

Quindlen, A. (1998). *Black and blue.* New York: Random House.

Sleeter, C. (2001). An analysis of the critiques of multicultural education. In J.A. Banks & C.A. McGee Banks (Eds.), *Handbook of research on multicultural education* (pp. 81-96). San Francisco: Jossey-Bass.

Stanford, A.F. (2003). *Bodies in a broken world: Women novelists of color & the politics of medicine.* Chapel Hill: University of North Carolina Press.

Wear, D. (2003). Insurgent multiculturalism: Rethinking how and why we teach culture in medical education. *Academic Medicine, 78*, 549-554.

West, C. (1992, August 2). Learning to talk of race. *New York Times Magazine, 141*, 24.

Williams, P.J. (1998). *Seeing a color-blind future: The paradox of race.* New York: Noonday Press.

Zais, R. (1976). *Curriculum: Principles and foundations.* New York: Thomas Y. Cromwell.

Chapter 6

YOU SAY SELF-INTEREST, I SAY ALTRUISM

Jack Coulehan
State University of New York at Stony Brook

H. L. Mencken taught us, "For every human problem, there is a neat, simple solution; and it is always wrong" (1990). This is an apt conclusion about the current project to instill more "professionalism" in medical education. The movement to teach and evaluate professionalism in medical training is likely to fail because the intervention is too simple, too neat, too flimsy, and does not fully engage the problems it attempts to address. These problems, as I conceive of them, are both internal and external to the profession. Internally, the community of medicine suffers from an impoverished moral imagination, and many of its practitioners suffer from existential conflict and timidity. Externally, the profession is beset on all sides by the disappointment, dissatisfaction, and misunderstanding of the people whom we are supposed to serve. So yes, professionalism in medicine does appear to be in bad shape these days; but no, Professionalism—with a capital "P" indicating the Simple Answer—will not revive it.

In this essay I present a series of reflections on today's culture of medicine and medical education, with particular emphasis on the V-word: virtue. I want to address the issue that Larry Churchill (1989) raised more than 15 years ago: "How did we get to this point of not valuing a distinctive professional ethic? A profession without its own distinctive moral convictions has nothing to profess." If indeed we have nothing to profess, then an aggressive program to instill and promote a code of professional behavior will be both artificial and bound for failure. In place of professionalism, I want to suggest a more comprehensive solution, in essence a rebirth of medical morality for the 21st century.

It is likely, however, that many readers will find these suggestions hopelessly naïve and unrealistic. But first, I provide a brief history of this most recent call for professionalism in medical education.

A RECENT HISTORY OF PROFESSIONALISM

As far as I can remember, "professionalism" was not a hot topic in medical education ten or fifteen years ago. Biomedical ethics, which focuses mostly on patient rights and the structure and process of shared decision making, had replaced old-fashioned professional ethics, which had dwelt on the special obligations of physicians (Beauchamp & Childress, 2001; Churchill, 1989; Jonsen, 1992; Jonsen, Siegler, & Winslade, 2002; Veatch, 1985). Professional ethics had acquired an unwarranted bad reputation as being more a set of rules to protect the interests of physicians than a code of moral conduct to protect patients. A few biomedical ethicists developed their new morality from the old vantage point of professional virtue (Coles, 1989; Drane, 1988; Pellegrino, 1985; Pellegrino, 1989; Pellegrino & Thomasma, 1993), but their works tended to lack the edge and bite of "hard" ethics and rarely served as the meat-and-potatoes of ethics teaching. In teaching about the "good" doctor, we made a distinction between talking about the way good doctors ought to behave (ethics courses) and walking the walk; i.e., following in the footsteps of good doctors. While virtue theory was amorphous and boring as an academic subject, we assumed that physicians-in-training would acquire professional values by osmosis from mentors and role models as they progressed through medical training, just as generations of physicians had presumably done in the past.

In 2005 the situation has changed dramatically. Today, the term "professionalism" is springing like kudzu from every nook and cranny of medical education. In the last few years, the American Association of Medical Colleges (AAMC), the Accreditation Council for Graduate Medical Education (ACGME), the American College of Physicians (ACP), and other organizations have generated major initiatives to teach professionalism as a core competency in medicine, and to require that educators use measurable indicators and outcomes to assess professionalism (AAMC, 2005; ACGME, 2005; ABIM, 2005; Barry, Cyran, & Anderson, 2000; Epstein & Hundert, 2002; Medical Professionalism Project, 2002).

Why the rapid change? To understand that, we need to consider the context, in particular the forces inside and outside of the profession that educators believe they need to respond to in order to create highly competent and ethical professionals who are equipped to deal with rapid scientific, social and economic change. Over the past several decades, U.S. medicine has evolved into a vast, increasingly expensive technological profit center, in which self-interest is easily conflated with altruism. Treatment becomes more efficacious but also more harmful than we can easily understand; physicians and patients grow increasingly dissatisfied; the system becomes incredibly expensive, yet remains inequitable and limited in scope; and a lingering cultural belief in relationship-based medical practice casts a pall over subspecialty and managed care practice. As these problems developed, medical educators responded by fashioning several generations of well-intended but ineffective solutions. Early innovations included creating the specialty of family medicine; propagating a so-called new paradigm—the biopsychosocial model; promoting generalism in education; instituting courses in biomedical ethics; and adopting problem-based learning in pre-clinical education. More recent innovations involved creating evidence-based medicine and putting considerably more effort into the theory and process of education, including core competencies, behavioral objectives, and 360-degree evaluation. Still, the situation was not improving; the *minds* of our students were sharper than ever, but their *hearts* appeared to be listless, and their moral compass kept drifting away. Then we came up with a new tack, a Next Wave in medical education—we would henceforth demand that professionalism be taught and our trainees be evaluated in their performance of professional behaviors. The stakes are high indeed: How To Make Students into Better Doctors and, indirectly, How To Improve American Medical Care.

Professionalism is "the conduct, aims, and qualities that characterize or mark a profession or professional person" (*The New Shorter Oxford English Dictionary*, 1993). This definition includes conduct (behavior), aims (motivation), and qualities (traits or virtues), not just one or another of these categories. Note, too, that these terms are not synonyms, but rather refer to different but intrinsically related aspects of human functioning. Conduct arises from aims, which, in turn, are conditioned by qualities. For young physicians to become more humane and effective healers, they need to demonstrate more appropriate professional conduct. But that is not possible unless their education also engages motivation and virtue.

My criticism of the new professionalism movement is that it focuses on skills and practices. According to this formulation, professionalism is a type of expertise that has been underrepresented in today's medical training. To remedy this problem, we need to take steps similar to those we use in teaching other forms of expertise. For example, we begin by listing requisite knowledge and skills. However, where do the items on this professionalism list come from? Ultimately, they derive from values and attitudes embedded in the tradition of medicine, as viewed now through a 21st century lens.

But the tradition of professional virtue cannot meaningfully be translated into expertise in the absence of two additional factors. First, the young physician must understand where these traditions, these Oaths, aphorisms, virtues, and quaint behaviors, came from. They have to be embedded in a system of understanding and meaning that is big enough and compelling enough to compete with contemporary hedonistic individualism on the one hand, and medicine as a purely technical enterprise on the other. Second, and this should be obvious, the young physician needs to take a version of this system of meaning and value to heart. In other words, becoming a physician involves a *conversion* and *witnessing*, not just the adoption of certain patterns of behavior. To the extent that today's professionalism focuses on expertise at the expense of understanding, conversion, and witnessing, the movement is an example of H. L. Mencken's neat and simple, but wrong, solution.

Next, we explore how this focus on expertise is translated into the medical curriculum.

THE STATE OF THE ART

The Two Cultures

Many observers have described a conflict between what we think we are teaching medical students and young physicians—the explicit or formal curriculum, and a second set of beliefs and values that they learn from other sources—the tacit, informal, or hidden curriculum (Bloom, 1989; Coulehan & Williams, 2001a, 2001b, 2003; Hafferty & Franks, 1994; Hundert, 1996; Rothman, 2000; Stephenson, Higgs, & Sugarman, 2001; Swick, Szenas, Danoff, Whitcomb, 1999; Wear, 1998; Wear & Castellani, 2000). This conflict begins during pre-clinical education, but becomes more pronounced and significant when they reach the hospital and clinic. As students and house officers wend their way through years of training, they gradually adopt the medical culture and its value system as their own. An important aspect of this socialization is the transfer of a set of beliefs and values regarding what it means to be a *good* physician, some of it dealt with explicitly in courses, classes, rounds, advice, or other teaching designed to instill professional values. For example, medical ethics and humanities courses may articulate the special moral obligations that arise in the physician-patient relationship, as well as the role of physicians in society.

Alternatively, tacit learning includes those aspects of learning and the socialization process that instill professional values and identity without explicitly articulating those issues. This "hidden" curriculum goes on continuously, day after day, throughout medical training. While the explicit curriculum focuses on empathy, communication, relief of suffering, trust, fidelity, and the patient's best interest, in the hospital environment these values are largely pushed aside by the tacit learning of objectivity, detachment, wariness, and distrust—distrust of emotions, patients, insurance companies, administrators, and the state.

Peter Williams and I have argued elsewhere that such conflict between tacit and explicit values seriously distorts medical professionalism (2001a, 2001b, 2003). At an experiential level, medical students and house officers attempt to relieve or resolve their internal conflict by adopting one of three styles of professional identity:

Some students and residents abandon traditional values and adopt a purely technical view of medical practice consistent with hospital culture. Thus, they tailor their conception of the "good" physician to fit their experience. They become cynical about duty, fidelity, confidentiality, and integrity. They question their own motivation and those of their patients and their patients' families. They adopt an objective professional identity that narrows their sphere of responsibility to the technical arena. Given this ethos, it would be quite reasonable to say: "He's an extremely good doctor, but he sure is nasty with patients." To those who subscribe to this ethic, being a "good" doctor is entirely a technical accomplishment.

Other students and residents internalize an identity of *non-reflective professionalism.* In this belief system, physicians consciously adhere to traditional medical values, while unconsciously basing their behavior, or some of it, on opposing values. Non-reflective professionalism is a type of self-delusion in which young physicians believe that when they act in accordance with tacit values they learned in the hospital, they actually manifest the explicit values they learned in the classroom. For example, hospital culture says that the most effective way to demonstrate compassion is to be detached and not get close to your patients. Similarly, hospital culture says that you best serve the patient's interest by substituting technological intervention for personal interaction. Because culturally we associate benefit with "doing everything" and "being aggressive," patients themselves tend to accept their physicians' predilection toward performing too many, rather than too few, interventions. In other words, non-reflective physicians could view themselves as engaging in patient advocacy while at the same time benefiting personally from the additional revenue this generates.

Finally, a third group of students and residents manage to overcome the conflict between tacit and explicit socialization and to emerge with genuine humanistic values that have coalesced into an altruistic professional persona. In our earlier papers, we speculated on factors that tend to protect or immunize students against the contamination of hospital culture and the tacit curriculum. The important point to make here is that many young physicians do, in fact, emerge from their training as professionals who are as good and as virtuous as can be.

Williams and I claimed that a large percentage of our graduates can best be characterized as non-reflective professionals; that is, physicians who sincerely believe they embody virtues like fidelity, self-effacement, integrity, compassion, and so forth, while acting in ways that conflict with these virtues and, in fact, acting in ways that contribute to contemporary problems in health care, such as rising costs, inadequate physician-patient communication, and widespread dissatisfaction. It is this group of physicians that most clearly exemplifies Albert Jonsen's (1983) insight about the core dynamic of professionalism: "The central paradox in medicine is the tension between self-interest and altruism."

HOSPITAL CULTURE

Clearly, the tension between self-interest and altruism is a fact of human nature that medical education ought to recognize and attempt to ameliorate. Thus far, I have used the term *hospital culture* in a rather non-narrative way, but before going on, I want to ask the reader to reflect on his or her own personal experience of the hospital milieu. Step into the units and halls of a contemporary teaching hospital. Listen to the conversations among physicians and between physicians and other health professionals. Listen to the words and silences between trainees and their attendings. Immerse yourself in the oral culture of modern hospital practice. Pay attention to the stories that people tell. What kinds of stories are they? Which stories are especially meaningful? Where does the energy lie? How do the stories fit together? In other words, in what sort of moral world does clinical medical education take place?

First, it seems apparent that the world is centered outside the patient room. It exists in hallways and conference rooms and unit stations. Generally, physicians enter patient rooms as little as possible. While inside the room, they tend to listen as little as possible. Their interaction with patients appears to play a remarkably small role in contributing to the "received wisdom" of hospital culture. In fact, procedures performed *on* patients are much more likely to be the starting place for the stories that doctors tell one another than are their conversations *with* patients.

Second, the stories that permeate the hospital ethos don't usually have patients as their protagonists, and often not even as ancillary characters that play human roles. Rather, patients quite frequently serve as clever or frustrating or even stupid plot devices—obstacles or challenges that impair the story's progress; or sometimes they may serve as positive plot devices, unexpected gifts that facilitate the story's successful resolution. The protagonists or heroes are usually doctors, although in an increasing percentage of cases the heroes may be cyborgs; i.e., machines of one sort or another, or complex, disembodied processes.

The stories tend to have a wider array of potential villains. In one with a straightforward plot, there may not even be a villain as such, but only an impersonal negative force—the disease, or some form of natural disaster. But in more complex cases, other health professionals may appear as quite satisfactory villains; e.g., the arrogant subspecialist, the power hungry surgeon, the incompetent nurse, the stupid medical student, and so forth. Moreover, the patient's own family may serve as a breeding ground for malevolence, villains as a result of being present (e.g., the hostile, questioning daughter) or being absent (e.g., the long-lost son in California). Finally, when patients do enter the stories as characters, they often do so as Bad Guys, with scripts that that demonstrate ignorance, anger, and—above all—non-compliance. Patients also play another important role in hospital stories—as the butt of gallows humor.

Third, a quick survey of the universe of hospital stories reveals that it is rather flat; not very vibrant or creative. However, it can be extremely stimulating from an intellectual perspective. Embedded within the stores are puzzles that can be extraordinarily complex; diagnostic dilemmas, complicated drug interactions, physiological conundrums. These quandaries share some characteristics with crossword puzzles (what is the correct label?), jigsaw puzzles (how does everything fit together?), and other games that require speed, endurance, and excellent hand-eye coordination. However, the stories remain flat because they contain little emotional resonance, and the characters are two-dimensional.

Fourth, the lack of emotional resonance in patient-and-doctor stories doesn't mean that hospital culture is unfeeling. It's just that most of the *recognized* feelings are those of doctors and other health professionals; and, however they are experienced internally, they tend to be expressed in negative ways; e.g., "This place sucks!" "That gomer in 1215 is a real pain in the ass." "I'm so pissed off at that resident." Although expressions like these are permissible, the ethos disapproves of emotion and favors stoic acceptance or whatever comes. This is one way that doctors demonstrate their superiority over patients, who often let their feelings get out of control.

Finally, as should be clear by this point, the virtues and values articulated in the stories that constitute hospital culture bear little relationship to the traditional ethos and morality of medicine: You say self-interest; I say altruism. You say the patient is an object of interest; I say the patient is a subject of respect. You say the bottom line is to free up the bed; I say the goal is to promote healing.

In presenting this thumbnail sketch of the world in which medical students and young physicians experience the "hidden" curriculum, I need to readily admit its limitations. First, these comments relate to the culture of medicine, and not to the cultures of nursing, social work, chaplaincy, or any other profession in the hospital. These cultures, of course, overlap, reverberate, and influence one another but—and this is quite remarkable—they seem to influence the culture of medicine very little. While physicians in the hospital are completely dependent upon multiple other professionals and support persons, medical culture remains rather isolated and uninfluenced by them, much to the dismay of others. The second limitation is equally important. I've dealt in broad strokes and generalizations. Fortunately, vibrant and edifying stories do exist, and many physicians and students recount them. It is by no means an entirely hostile culture and, as described in earlier paragraphs, many trainees manage to "graduate" from it with positive professional identities.

ANOTHER VIEW OF THE STATE OF THE ART

In 2003 Thomas Inui published a report entitled "A Flag in the Wind: Educating for Professionalism in Medicine" based on his six months as scholar-in-residence at the AAMC. Inui studied the extensive literature on professionalism and conducted interviews and focus groups, leavened, I am sure, by his own long experience as a physician and medical educator. In the following, I quote the full text of his eight conclusions about teaching professionalism because they provide the most accurate and concise summary I have seen of the "state of the art" in medical education.

The major elements of what most of us in medicine mean by professionalism have been described well, not once but many times.

Among these descriptions, there is a high degree of congruence, probably because our general understanding of the attributes of a *virtuous person* serves as a foundation for our thinking about the needed qualities of the trustworthy medical professional.

What the literature and rhetoric of medicine lacks is a clear recognition of the *gap* between these widely recognized manifestations of virtue in action and *what we actually do* in the circumstances in which we live our lives.

We may be unconscious of some of this gap, but even when conscious we are silent or inarticulate about the dissonance and, in our silence, do not assist our students to understand our challenges when attempting to live up to our profession's ideals.

In the process of becoming medical professionals themselves, our students learn powerfully from the systems in which we work and what they see us do (the hidden and informal curriculum), not only from what they hear us say (the formal curriculum).

Under present circumstances, students become cynical about the profession of medicine—indeed, may see cynicism as intrinsic to medicine—because they see us "say one thing and do another."

Additional courses on medical professionalism are unlikely to fundamentally alter this regrettable circumstance. Instead, we will actually have to change our behaviors, our institutions, and ourselves.

The opportunities for change that will enhance the modeling of medical professionalism are myriad, but the most difficult challenge of all may be the need to understand—and to be explicitly mindful of, and articulate about—medical education as a special form of personal and professional formation that is rooted in the daily activities of individuals and groups in academic medical communities. (Inui, 2003)

Inui recognizes that the gap between belief and behavior that characterizes the faculty and staff of our teaching hospitals is at least partly unconscious (conclusion #4). To the extent that the gap is unconscious, these physicians manifest *non-reflective professionalism*; that is, in their professional formation they internalized the belief that certain non-virtuous behaviors are virtuous, since they are "the way things are in medicine." For example, the best way to care for the patient (and thus demonstrate altruism and benevolence) is to perform actions that also benefit the hospital, or the medical service, or the radiology department, etc. because each of these institutions serves as a kind of prerequisite for patient care. Likewise, the term "care" must be understood as a package of specific (billable) services because that is, to the non-reflective professional, the only way to operationalize the amorphous concept of caring. Thus, these attending physicians justify dehumanizing and alienating aspects of hospital culture as, in fact, being for the patient's benefit, and they teach this to their students and residents.

The term "non-reflective" suggests that these physicians simply never step back and consider the impact of their behavior on themselves and others, especially patients. Their primary concern is the impact of their behavior on more objective end-points, like disease, or data collection, or getting the day's work done. Thus, they need not be aware of the discrepancy between their avowed values and, let's say, their lack of attention to their patients' fears and pain. However, as Inui's conclusion implies, another part of the institutional gap between belief and practice is probably conscious and, therefore, hypocritical. Some physicians simply don't care that much about patients as persons, but they do care about basic research or biomedical technology. When these physicians are forced to teach, and thus serve as representatives of professional virtue, they behave hypocritically. Trainees detect this and respond by becoming cynical (conclusion #6).

When Inui argues that "additional courses on medical professionalism are unlikely to fundamentally alter this regrettable circumstance. . . . We will actually have to change our behaviors, our institutions, and our selves" (conclusion #7), he expresses why professionalism *as a set of concepts or rules or objectives* will not have an impact on medical education. To improve the quality of our students' professional formation, we must begin by changing ourselves, and hence our behaviors, and ultimately our institutions. Only then will we be in a position to mold our students' professional virtue. A White Coat Ceremony simply won't suffice.

But what sort of change is required? What motivates people to adopt the underlying values of medical professionalism? As Inui observes, the endpoint is neither mysterious nor controversial. In fact, there is widespread agreement about the characteristics a virtuous physician should have (conclusions #1 and #2). In the following paragraphs I want to sketch the origins of medical virtues, with the intent of showing that they arise ultimately from a series of cultural narratives. For them to be meaningful in practice, the person—the professional—must adopt them as part of his or her own narrative. Virtues are not abstractions; they arise from stories.

PROFESSIONALISM AND PROFESSIONAL VIRTUES: ORIGINS IN THREE TRADITIONS

The Hippocratic Tradition

The tradition of medical professionalism holds that there are deeply held values internal to the goals of the profession, a commitment to moral behavior grounded in "that which I hold most sacred" (to quote a contemporary version of the Hippocratic Oath), and, as a result of sharing these values and beliefs, a strong sense of community identity. Values, beliefs, and community are arguably characteristics of religion, as well as of professionalism, especially when pursued in the name of the "most sacred." In practice, the traditional view of medical professionalism exists as a kind of narrative ideal that developed over 2,500 years as a summation of, and reflection upon, the stories of actual physicians in different times and cultures. I'd like to call this perspective *narrative-based professionalism*, in contrast to *rule-based professionalism*, which is the term I'll use to lump (perhaps unfairly) the recent emphasis on professionalism as described above, which is bound as a set of rules, objectives, competencies, or measurable behaviors.

Western physicians generally accept the Hippocratic tradition as the core of medical morality. The Oath contains three parts. It specifies duties to one's colleagues, teachers, and the profession as a whole; e.g., keep the precepts secret, treat your colleagues as family, and perpetuate the art by teaching the next generation. It lists duties to one's patients; e.g., benefit them, keep their confidences, and avoid having sex with them, or prescribing deadly drugs.

The third part of this tradition is the act of professing or witnessing the commitment. Originally, aspirants swore by Apollo, Aesculapius, and various other gods of healing. Nowadays, we've dumped the gods and in the version we use at Stony Brook the student swears *"by all that I hold most sacred."* Notice, however, one's public *profession* depends for its moral efficacy on the oath-taker's integrity (i.e., bearing false witness is immoral) and also on the assumption that the oath-taker *does* hold something "most sacred." But what if the individual doesn't hold anything sacred? Or has never given serious consideration to the meaning of "sacred"? Or what if the most important value in the young physician's life is getting ahead, making money, or becoming a famous scientist?

Still, in some ways the more we learn about Hippocratic physicians, the more we are able to visualize ourselves in them. They believed that diseases are natural and predictable, and we can learn to understand them by experience and systematic observation, Moreover, the Hippocratic physicians were practical tradesmen, committed to earning a living, as well as to mastering the healing art. However, they were convinced of the close relationship between professional morality and mastery of the healing art, as the Hippocratic *Precepts* expresses, "For where there is love of man, there is also love of the art" (Lloyd, 1984.) And, of course, in the *Epidemics,* the most widely (if incorrectly) quoted Hippocratic saying: "As to diseases, make a habit of two things—to help, or at least to do no harm" (Lloyd, 1984).

However, in other ways these physicians do not live up to our received image of virtuous doctoring. The Hippocratic physician had no general duty to treat sick and vulnerable people. If a doctor accepted a patient, yes, of course, he was obligated to do his best to benefit that patient. But the decision to accept a patient was a practical matter based on prognosis, ethnicity, social status, and ability to pay. Thus, a doctor might turn down a terminal case because his reputation would suffer when the patient died. Likewise, there was no obligation to care for slaves, or for those who could not afford one's services. Hippocratic virtues included honor and integrity, but not necessarily respect or compassion, especially for inferior groups like slaves, barbarians, and women.

The Religious Tradition

The Common Era brought an infusion of religious values that transformed and deepened Greek and Roman medical virtues, bringing renewed energy into medical professionalism. With the dissemination of Judaism, Christianity, and Islam throughout the Western world, new values and virtues were superimposed on the earlier ones. The monotheistic God demanded a stronger and more wide-reaching morality than the Greek and Roman deities he replaced. These narratives placed high value on virtues like compassion, benevolence, and self-sacrifice. In Christendom, St. Luke's story of the Good Samaritan became a model for the virtuous physician (Luke. 10: 25-41). The 13th century Prayer of Moses Maimonides reflects Medieval Christian, Islamic, and Jewish values: "Do not allow thirst for profit, ambition for renown and admiration, to interfere with my profession, for these are the enemies of truth and of love for mankind and they can lead astray in the great task of attending to the welfare of thy creatures" (Friedenwald, 1917). Similarly, the modern Oath of Islamic Physicians expresses the commitment to be "an instrument of God's mercy, extending my medical care to near and far, virtuous and sinner and friend and enemy" (Physicians for Human Rights, 2005). We continue to value compassion and caring, a commitment to helping the needy, and the ideal of humanistic education, even though they may no longer be grounded in religious practice.

The Enlightenment Tradition

The Enlightenment brought additional depth to the professional tradition, particularly in the realm of relationships, such as the concepts of empathy (albeit under different terminology), the physician-patient contract, and the therapeutic role of the physician-patient interaction. This tradition was first summarized by the Manchester physician Thomas Percival in his *Medical Ethics* of 1803, a book of precepts and rules thoroughly grounded in contemporary Scottish philosophical thought (Leake, quoted in Baker, 1993), especially John Gregory's 1772 *Lectures on the Duties and Qualifications of a Physician* (McCullough, 1998) and David Hume's theory of the sentiments (Morris, 2005). Percival develops a moral psychology based on Hume's concept of *sympathy,* i.e., the trait that allows us to form an idea of another person's character, resulting in a "mental impression" that matches the feeling the other person experiences. To use more modern terms, while "sympathy" may perhaps be the psychological basis for compassion, the skill involved in "forming an impression that matches the feeling the other person experiences" is nowadays called *empathy* or *clinical empathy*, and is the focus of considerable interest and investigation in medicine (Bennett, 2001; Connelly, 1998; Coulehan, 1996, 1997, 1999; Coulehan, Platt, Frankl, Salazar, Lown, & Fox, 2001; More & Milligan, 1994).

From this perspective, Percival developed the basis for the modern concept of relationship-based medicine. Of 72 precepts in his chapters that deal with medical practice, 57 are concerned with doctor-patient interactions. For the first time, patient-as-person appears to be an integral part of the professional ethos; for example, in the precept, "The feelings and emotions of the patients, under critical circumstances, require to be known and to be attended to, no less than the symptoms of their diseases" (Leake, quoted in Baker, 1993). Enlightenment professional ethics continued the tradition of deriving professional values from a broader conceptual context, in this case the Christian virtues. The good physician must be knowledgeable, compassionate, sympathetic, temperate, sober, committed to education and self-improvement, and ready to acknowledge error.

WHAT NEEDS TO BE DONE

To reiterate, professionalism in its current educational manifestation retains (or modifies) many rules and guidelines and codes of behavior derived from the tradition of medical virtue, but it avoids grappling with deep issues of value and character formation and fails to internalize the narrative tradition of medicine. In essence, today's professionalism is something like a Walt Disney version of a work of literature. In no way does it address the fact that in medicine formation of character is as important as technical education (Pellegrino, 1989). To seriously address formation of character, medical education needs to live and breathe and *believe* professional values. To begin this process, my colleagues and I suggested four major educational initiatives (Coulehan, Platt, Frankel, Salazar, Lown, & Fox, 2001; Coulehan & Williams, 2003), none of which is particularly innovative and all of which overlap a great deal. Perhaps the only new aspect of this proposal is the determination *not* to be modest or "practical" about what can be achieved.

Role modeling

The first requirement for a sea change in professionalism is to increase dramatically the number of role model physicians at every stage of medical education. By role model physicians I mean full-time faculty members who exemplify professional virtue in their interactions with patients, staff, and trainees; who have a broad, humanistic perspective; and who are devoted to teaching and willing to forego high income in order to teach. Because such role model physicians are reflective, as opposed to non-reflective, in their professionalism, their presence would dilute and diminish the conflict between tacit and explicit values, especially in the hospital and clinic. The teaching environment would contain fewer hidden messages that say "Detach" while at the same time overt messages are saying "Engage." What trainees need is time and humanism. However, role model faculty cannot fully pay for themselves. Therefore, we need major new investment in financing medical education.

Self-awareness curriculum

Another prerequisite for developing narrative professionalism is to provide throughout medical school and residency a safe venue for students and residents to share experiences and enhance personal awareness. Doctors need to understand their own beliefs, feelings, attitudes, and response patterns. One of the earliest proponents of this view was the British psychiatrist Michael Balint (1972), who focused attention on the therapeutic power of the physician-patient interaction with his aphorism, "The doctor is the drug." Balint encouraged physicians to meet regularly in small groups to discuss their difficulties with patients and their personal reactions to practice. Physicians tend to avoid emotions, identifying them as negative, and often confusing knowledge of a feeling with the experience of that feeling. They are particularly vulnerable to feelings of anxiety, loneliness, frustration, anger, depression, and helplessness when caring for chronically, seriously, and terminally ill patients. They cope with these emotions in ineffectual ways, often by attempting to suppress them. The more physicians reverse this process by developing an understanding of their own beliefs, attitudes, and feelings, the more likely they will be able to connect with, and respond to, their patients' experience (Branch et al., 1995; Branch et al., 2001; Pololi, Frankel, Clay, & Jobe, 2000; Novack et al., 1997; Meier, Back, & Morrison, 2001; Farber, Novack, & O'Brien, 1997).

In addition, the trainee's ethical development may be hindered by everyday learning situations. These include conflicts between the requirements of medical education and those of good patient care, assignments that entail responsibility exceeding the student's capabilities, and personal involvement in substandard care. Once again, the opportunity to discuss, analyze, critique, and sometimes repair these experiences allows students to find their own voice and may eventually empower them to use their voice effectively.

Community service

To instill professional values, the medical curriculum must include socially relevant service-oriented learning. Interaction with patients in the hospital or office setting is insufficient to convert students to a sense of stewardship social responsibility. The AMA Code (in VII) specifies, "A physician shall recognize a responsibility to participate in activities contributing to an improved community." In another section (III) the Code indicates, "A physician shall . . . recognize a responsibility to seek changes in (legal) requirements which are contrary to the best interests of the patient"

(AMA Council on Ethical and Judicial Affairs, 2005). If these requirements are important manifestations of professionalism, they need to be addressed in medical education. For example, students might select from a menu of service-oriented educational activities, e.g., HIV education in local high schools, volunteer work in hospices, health services for migrant workers, or environmental or other politically active volunteer organizations.

Narrative competence

Medical practice is structured around narrative. However, as a result of the tension between explicit and tacit values, even though medicine is a narrative-rich environment, students learn to objectify their patients and devalue the subjective. As I illustrated earlier, today's hospital narratives, although they tend to be cynical, arrogant, egotistic, self-congratulatory, and highly rationalized while simultaneously suppressing and distorting human feelings, are nonetheless very influential in the formation of the professional persona. They are the narratives we have, but medical culture encourages us to see them as facts of life rather than as stories we've chosen to tell ourselves. Moreover, the student immersed in these stories has little time to listen to, and lacks the skill to understand, patient narratives or narratives of role model physicians.

Another prerequisite for renewed professionalism is the development of narrative competence, or "the ability to acknowledge, absorb, interpret, and act on the stories and plights of others" (Charon, 2001a). The narrative medicine movement is a way of reframing much of the knowledge and skills of good doctoring under the aegis of language, culture, and story (Charon, 2001a, 2001b; Greenhalgh & Hurwitz, 1998; Frank, 1995; Montgomery, 1991; Morris, 1998, 2001; Nelson, 1997). Students may enhance their repertoire of life experience and their assortment of role models by exposure to narratives of real and fictional physicians, and they may increase their understanding of their own developing professional identities by reflecting upon and writing about their experiences. (Bolton, 1999; Charon, 2001a; Coulehan & Clary, in press). In addition to writing and reflecting on their own experience, students may broaden and deepen their narrative competence though curricula that include biographies, memoirs, nonfictional medical accounts, medical and nonmedical fiction, poetry, and film. Through such stories, a student may vicariously gain access not just to the outward behavior and explicit advice of the physician, but also to the internal material—feelings, hopes, doubts, fears, questions, and ambiguities—that constitutes a narrated character's professional ethos. These narratives bring many living and breathing physician characters into the room, including negative representations that can serve as counter-models against which students may construct their own professional identities.

NARRATIVES OF PROFESSIONAL VIRTUE

I want to conclude by demonstrating the way in which fictional narratives can contribute to all four components of the "character formation" educational package just described. Obviously, studying creative literature plays only a small role in professional character formation. Nonetheless, it can serve to broaden the student's range of role models, to enhance self-awareness, to stimulate social responsibility, and to expand and deepen the student's narrative competence. In the following examples, I want to touch on how three short stories I frequently teach might help medical students understand the difference between rule-based and narrative-based approaches to professionalism.

In Mikhail Bulgakov's "The Steel Windpipe," a young physician with hardly any experience finds himself in charge of a small community hospital (Bulgakov, 2001). One of his first patients is a young girl brought to the hospital by her mother and grandmother. She is terrified because she can't breathe. The doctor quickly ascertains that the girl suffers from diphtheria, which has progressed to the point of near-total tracheal obstruction. He struggles to maintain a calm demeanor despite the anger he feels at the patient's mother and grandmother, who waited five days before bringing the child to the hospital for treatment.

With his patient on the verge of death, the doctor decides that only an emergency tracheotomy can save her. But there are two problems. First, the grandmother distrusts doctors and violently opposes surgery; she convinces the mother not to consent. In response to her refusal, the young physician completely loses his cool. He denounces the grandmother's advice, threatens the mother with her child's death, and finally begs her to agree to the tracheotomy. The second problem is that the doctor actually realizes that he is in way over his head. Despite his insistence on aggressive care, he has never performed the procedure and is afraid that he might kill the girl if he attempts a tracheotomy. Nonetheless, under his intense pressure the mother finally agrees, and the doctor quickly performs the surgery and inserts a tracheostomy tube ("steel windpipe"). The outcome is marvelous: the little girl breathes freely; her crisis passes; her life is saved.

"The Steel Windpipe" is a classic tale of the doctor-as-savior (Monroe & Coulehan, 2002). In many years of teaching this story to first year medical students, I've rarely encountered one who wasn't stirred by the hero's performance. These future physicians find it easy to visualize themselves performing such heroic acts. They see themselves as doing whatever it takes to save their patients' lives, even if involves the "tough love" of breaking rules and battering parental superstition. Of course, as their clinical training proceeds, this romantic vision quickly fades. Nonetheless, pre-clinical students respond to "The Steel Windpipe" and to other, similar Bulgakov stories like "Baptism by Rotation" and "The Embroidered Towel" with unbridled enthusiasm. They realize intuitively that heroic action requires the whole person, that it takes more than mere technical training to resolve a crisis. The physician also needs integrity, courage, quick thinking, and the ability to function in the face of conflict, pressure, and strong emotion.

But how professional is the behavior of Bulgakov's young doctor? Does he act like a responsible physician in saving this little girl's life? He would perhaps remain a hero if we transferred him from a hospital in Revolutionary Russia to a contemporary episode of *ER* on television, although we might expect some muttering in the background about him being a "loose cannon." But how would his behavior be judged in a real-life emergency room? Does he demonstrate medical professionalism? Well, yes and no. The doctor in "The Steel Windpipe" demonstrates courage, decisiveness, beneficence, and compassion. However, he bombs-out with regard to prudence, and he is disrespectful of his patient's mother and grandmother. He allows his anger to show, uses coercive techniques to obtain consent, and undertakes a procedure that he is inadequately trained to perform. If the tracheotomy had gone wrong, or the girl had died in spite of it, we could just as well use the story to illustrate the danger of such unprofessional behavior as overstepping one's level of competence and using coercive techniques to obtain consent.

Thus, the doctor demonstrates virtues we tend to value highly in urgent medical situations, but he also runs roughshod over many of the rules of professionalism. Let me contrast Bulgakov's hero with another physician from Russian literature. In Anton Chekhov's short story called "Darkness," a distraught peasant approaches a rural doctor to beg for a favor (Chekhov, 1887/2003). The man's brother was sent to prison for breaking into a bakery. There were extenuating circumstances: the brother was drunk at the time and didn't mean any harm. Could the doctor use his influence to get the man's brother released? At first, the doctor explains that he has no influence over the legal system; there is simply nothing he can do. However, the peasant won't give up. He hounds the doctor until the latter becomes so enraged he slams the door in the man's face.

Medical students find this fictional physician despicable. They immediately point out his insensitivity, arrogance, dismissiveness, and lack of empathy. However, when one looks carefully at the question of his professionalism, the answer is not so straightforward. First of all, the doctor does take the time to speak to this man who approaches him on the street. Secondly, he is truthful—in fact, medical doctors do *not* have power over the judiciary—and he also provides a reasonable suggestion, i.e., that the man take his request to the district court. Finally, neither the supplicant nor his brother is this particular doctor's identified patient. In fact, Chekhov's doctor adheres to most of the relevant canons of professionalism, except in the end when he becomes angry at his supplicant's persistence. So why do the students have such a negative reaction?

For one thing, although the doctor in "Darkness" obeys the rules, he does not demonstrate the kind of virtue we like to see in our doctors. He fails to act in a recognizably compassionate manner. He refuses to advocate for this poor ignorant fellow who, after all, has petitioned him for help. (Some may even feel that the fact of their speaking together constitutes the initiation of a doctor-patient relationship.) And finally, when the doctor eventually gets angry, he acts in an abrupt and arrogant manner. We don't like the character, but yet it is difficult to specify precisely what is unprofessional in his behavior.

The students' responses to these two fictional physicians serve to illustrate a difficulty with using rule-based professionalism as the standard for medical virtue and, consequently, with the attempt to re-energize (or re-humanize) medical education by introducing explicit professionalism curricula. The current program begins by setting forth lists of behavioral norms for physicians; the norms are drawn from professional ethics, which, in turn, is based on a mixture of tradition, social etiquette, religious values, and philosophy, primarily virtue theory; in essence, a comprehensive moral vision of medicine. For the sake of argument, let's say that the new professionalism movement depends very heavily on the lists and is very light on the comprehensive moral vision. In this case students will find that the program lacks energy and feels rather sterile to them. But because they are pragmatists, they will adopt the rules and get on with their careers. This form of competency-based professionalism may well produce doctors who know and obey the professional rules but, like Chekhov's character in "Darkness," don't embody the true spirit of professionalism. Following the rules does not necessarily make a good (or humane or admirable) physician.

However, if you define professionalism as a more comprehensive moral vision of medicine, for example, the virtue-based moralities of medicine developed by Pellegrino and Thomasma (1993), Drane (1988, 2003), Sulmasy (1997) and Coles (1989, 2000) rather than simply as a set of rules, you run into another problem. You attribute various virtues or attributes to "good" doctors; for example, the good doctor has integrity, compassion, courage, fidelity, humility, and so forth. To be a good doctor, the trainee must develop these virtues, so the professionalism curriculum is needed to facilitate that process. But how? How do we teach the virtues in medical school? And if it is possible to teach them, how much (what quantity of) of a given virtue is required before the trainee can be considered sufficiently virtuous? Let's say compassion and beneficence are virtues that predispose me to advocate for my patients, a posture that in some cases will demand that I put the patients' best interests before my own. Thus, these virtues do have behavioral consequences that we can measure; e.g., advocating for a patient with an insurance bureaucrat, or spending extra time with an anxious patient when you could have gone home for supper. But how much advocacy is enough? Or how many hours are enough? It isn't clear whether we can structure medical education to teach virtue, but even if we can, I doubt if reasonable physicians could all agree on the "target" levels of virtuousness.

Bulgakov implies a connection between the character of the newly minted physician and his successful intervention to save the child. The safe path would have been a more conventional, less risky, course of treatment. If he had then lost the patient, the death would have occurred within the safe haven of an established protocol. He would have gotten through the Morbidity & Mortality conference with flying colors. But the doctor put his self-esteem as well as his reputation on the line for the benefit of the little girl, a course that exposed her to significant risk. He was successful, but what if she had died in any case? In some ways this is a clear example of character versus rules.

But a character fault, perhaps even a serious one, need not *necessarily* prevent a person from being a good doctor. Again let's use a character from a short story to illustrate this point. In Susan Mates' "The Good Doctor" (1994) middle aged Dr. Helen van Horne has devoted her career to unselfishly caring for poor persons who otherwise lack access to medical care. For many years she practiced in rural East Africa; more recently, she serves as Chief of the Department of Medicine at City Hospital in South Bronx. Van Horne is a tough, no-nonsense woman who evidently gave up the comforts of marriage and family to devote herself to her profession.

While the patients in South Bronx initially dismiss her as another white do-gooder, they soon learn to respect her as a model of rectitude, dedication, and compassion. The Hispanic chief resident at City Hospital finds her an ideal role model.

Nonetheless, Dr. van Horne has an Achilles' heel. Her inner yearning for human comfort and sexual gratification draws her into intimate sexual contact with a lazy, irresponsible, but charming male medical student, who intends to "use" her to pass his clerkship. As a result Dr. van Horne first tells the failing student that she will give him the passing grade he doesn't deserve, but later she realizes the extent of her weakness and allows his actual grade to be recorded.

Medical students' responses to this story vary. A few students latch tightly to Dr. van Horne's egregious behavior, i.e., having sex with her student, condemn her for that, and then generalize to impugn the motivation for her life's work. In their opinion she isn't really courageous, compassionate, and altruistic; she is really a power-junkie, who "gets off" on lording it over the less fortunate. This cynical viewpoint, or at least a milder version of it, is widespread in our society. We apparently love to poke holes in any virtuous edifice (or person) we come across and, thereby, provoke a scandal; for example, MOTHER THERESA DISCOVERED TO HAVE SMOKED CIGARETTES!!!

The majority of students, however, take a more nuanced approach. They agree that Dr. van Horne has generally been a good person and a good physician, but they struggle with the implications of her recent peccadillo. How reflective was it of her overall character? What kind of relationships might she have had with subordinates in the past? On other occasions might she have performed unethical actions when influenced by someone preying on her lack or companionship and loneliness? "The Good Doctor" presents a more complicated picture of character than either of the earlier stories. It illustrates that virtue and character interact with, and are ways of looking at, the texture of one's personal narrative, rather than being separate and unchanging qualities.

CONCLUSIONS

Professionalism is *au courant* in medicine today, but the concept has a variety of sources and meanings. The movement to teach and evaluate professionalism in medical education presents somewhat of a conundrum. Its intent is laudable: to produce humanistic and virtuous physicians who, as such, will be better able to cope with and overcome the dehumanizing features of our health care system. However, its actual impact on medical education is likely to be small and perhaps misleading. Since educational initiatives must nowadays be judged by measurable outcome parameters, professionalism curricula focus on lists of rules physicians ought to follow and behaviors they should demonstrate. While such curricula often include references to virtues and personal qualities, these are in a sense peripheral to the teaching and learning because their impact cannot be specifically assessed.

Today's culture of medicine tends to be hostile to altruism, compassion, integrity, fidelity, self-effacement, and other traditional qualities. In fact, hospital culture, and the narratives that support it, implicitly identifies a very different set of professional qualities as "good," and sometimes these qualities are diametrically opposed to virtues that we explicitly teach. Students and young physicians experience internal conflict as they try to reconcile the explicit and covert or hidden curricula, and in the process of character formation they often develop non-reflective professionalism. Additional courses on professionalism are unlikely to alter this process. Instead, I propose a more comprehensive approach to changing the culture of medical education and to addressing the "central paradox in medicine," which is the "tension between self-interest and altruism" (Jonsen, 1983).

REFERENCES

Accreditation Council for Graduate Medical Education. (2001). *Outcome project.* Retrieved March 1, 2005, from the ACGME website: http://www.acgme.org/Outcome/

American Association of Medical Colleges. (2005). *Assessment of professionalism project.* Retrieved March 1, 2005, from the AAMC website: http://www.aamc.org/members/gea/professionalism.pdf

American Board of Internal Medicine. (2001). *Project professionalism.* Retrieved March 1, 2005 from the ABIM website: http://www.abim.org/pdf/profess.pdf

American Medical Association Council on Ethical and Judicial Affairs. (2004). *Code of medical ethics.* Retrieved March 1, 2005, from the AMA website: http://www.ama-assn.org/ama/pub/category/2512.html

Baker, R., (1993). Deciphering Percival's code. In R. Baker, D. Porter & R. Porter (Eds.), *The codification of medical morality* (pp. 196). Netherlands: Kluwer Academic Publishers.

Balint, M. (1972). *The doctor, his patient, and the illness.* New York: International Universities Press.

Barry, D., Cyran, E., & Anderson, R.J. (2000). Common issues in medical professionalism: Room to grow. *American Journal of Medicine, 108,* 136-142.

Beauchamp, T.L., & Childress, J.R. (2001). *Principles of biomedical ethics* (5th edition). New York: Oxford University Press.

Bennett, M.J. (2001). *The empathic healer: An endangered species?* New York: Academic Press.

Bloom, S.M. (1989). The medical school as a social organization: The sources of resistance to change. *Medical Education, 23,* 228-241.

Bolton, G. (1999). Stories at work: Reflective writing for practitioners. *The Lancet, 354,* 243-245.

Branch, W.T., Pels, R.J., Harper, G., Calkins, D., Forrow, L., & Mandell, F., et al. (1995). A new educational approach for supporting the professional development of third year medical students. *Journal of General Internal Medicine, 10*(12), 691-694.

Branch, W.T., Kern, D., Haidet, P., Weissmann, P., Gracey, C.F., Mitchell, G., et al. (2001). Teaching the human dimensions of care in clinical settings. *Journal of the American Medical Association, 286,* 1067-1074.

Bulgakov, M. (2001). The steel windpipe. In R. Reynolds & J. Stone (Eds.), *On doctoring* (3rd edition) (pp. 78-85). New York: Simon & Schuster.

Charon, R. (2001a). Narrative medicine. A model for empathy, reflection, profession, and trust. *Journal of the American Medical Association, 286,* 1897-1902.

Charon, R. (2001b). Narrative medicine: Form, function, and ethics. *Annals of Internal Medicine, 134,* 83-87.

Chekhov, A. (2003). Darkness. In J. Coulehan (Ed.), *Chekhov's doctors* (pp. 30-40). Kent, OH: Kent State University Press.

Churchill, L.R. (1989). Reviving a distinctive medical ethic. *The Hastings Center Report, 19*(3), 28-34.

Coles, R. (1989). *The call of stories: Teaching and the moral imagination.* Boston: Houghton Mifflin.

Coles, R. (2000). *Lives of moral leadership.* New York: Random House.

Connelly, J. (1998). Emotions, ethics, and decisions in primary care. *Journal of Clinical Ethics,9,* 225-234.

Coulehan, J.L. (1996). Tenderness and steadiness: Emotions in medical practice. *Literature and Medicine, 14,* 222-236.

Coulehan, J.L. (1997). Being a physician. In M.B. Mengel & W.L. Holleman (Eds.), *Fundamentals of clinical practice: A textbook on the patient, doctor, and society* (pp. 73-101). New York: Plenum Publishing Company.

Coulehan, J. (1999). An alternative view: Listening to patients. *The Lancet, 354,* 1467-1468.

Coulehan, J., & Clary, P. (in press). Healing the healer: Poetry in palliative care. *Journal of Palliative Care.*

Coulehan, J., & Williams, P.C. (2001a). Professional ethics and social activism: Where have we been? Where are we going? In D. Wear & J. Bickel (Eds.), *Educating for professionalism: Creating a climate of humanism in medical education* (pp. 49-69). Iowa City: University of Iowa Press.

Coulehan, J., & Williams, P.C. (2001b). Vanquishing virtue: The impact of medical education. *Academic Medicine, 76,* 598-605.

Coulehan, J., & Williams, P.C. (2003). Conflicting professional values in medical education. *Cambridge Quarterly of Healthcare Ethics, 12,* 7-20.

Coulehan, J.L., Platt, F.W., Frankl, R., Salazar, W., Lown, B., & Fox, L. (2001). Let me see if I have this right: Words that build empathy. *Annuals of Internal Medicine, 135,* 221-227.

Drane, J.F. (1988). *Becoming a good doctor: The place of virtue and character in medical ethics.* Kansas City: Sheed & Ward.

Drane, J. (2003). *More human medicine: A liberal Catholic bioethics.* Edinboro, PA: Edinboro University Press.

Edelstein, L. (Trans.). (1943). From the Hippocratic oath: Text, translation, and interpretation. Baltimore: Johns Hopkins Press. Retrieved March 1, 2005 from the Dalhousie University, Kellogg Library's website: http://www.library.dal.ca/kellogg/Bioethics/codes/hippocraticoath.htm.

Epstein, R.M., & Hundert, E.M. (2002). Defining and assessing professional competence. *Journal of the American Medical Association, 287,* 226-235.

Farber, N.J., Novack, D.H., & O'Brien, M.K. (1997). Love, boundaries, and the patient physician relationship. *Archives of Internal Medicine, 157,* 2291-2294.

Frank, A.W. (1995). *The wounded storyteller: Body, illness, and ethics.* Chicago: University of Chicago Press.

Friedenwald, H. (Trans.). (1917). Prayer of Maimonides. *Bulletin of the Johns Hopkins Hospital, 28,* 260-261. Retrieved March 1, 2005 from the Dalhousie University, Kellogg Library's Website: http://www.library.dal.ca/kellogg/Bioethics/codes/maimonides.htm

Greenhalgh, T., & Hurwitz, B. (Eds.). (1998). *Narrative based medicine: Dialogue and discourse in clinical practice.* London: BMJ Books.

Hafferty, F.W., & Franks, R. (1994). The hidden curriculum, ethics teaching, and the structure of medical education. *Academic Medicine, 69,* 861-871.

Hundert, E.M. (1996). Characteristics of the informal curriculum and trainee's ethical choices. *Academic Medicine, 71,* 624-633.

Inui, T.S. (2003). *A flag in the wind: Educating for professionalism in medicine.* Washington, DC: Association of American Medical Colleges.

Jonsen, A.R. (1983).Watching the doctor. *New England Journal of Medicine, 308,* 1531-5.

Jonsen, A.R. (1992). *The new medicine and the old ethics.* Cambridge: Harvard University Press.

Jonsen, A.R., Siegler, M., & Winslade, W.J. (2002). *Clinical ethics.* New York: Macmillan Publishing Company.

Leake, C.D. (Ed.). (1927). *Percival's medical ethics.* New York: Williams and Wilkins.

Lloyd,G.E.R. (1984). *The writings of Hippocrates.* New York: Penguin Books.

Mates, S.O. (1994). The good doctor. In *The Good Doctor* (pp. 30-41). Iowa City: University of Iowa Press.

McCullough, L.B. (Ed.). (1998). *John Gregory and the invention of professional medical ethics and the profession of medicine* (Philosophy and Medicine, 57). Boston: Kluwer Academic.

Medical Professionalism Project. (2002). Medical professionalism in the new millennium: a physicians' charter. *The Lancet, 359,* 520-522.

Meier, D.E., Back, A.L., & Morrison, R.S. (2001). The inner life of physicians and care of the seriously ill. *Journal of the American Medical Association, 286,* 3007-3014.

Mencken, H. L., & Alstair Cooke (compiler). (1990). Mencken's metalaw. In *The vintage Mencken.* New York: Vintage.

Monroe, W., & Coulehan, J. (2002). Literature and medicine. In M.B. Mengel & W. L. Holleman (Eds.), *Fundamentals of clinical practice: A textbook on the patient, doctor, and society* (pp. 99-117). New York: Plenum Medical Books Company.

More, E.S., & Milligan, M.A. (Eds.). (1994). *The empathic practitioner: Empathy, gender, and medicine.* New Brunswick: Rutgers University Press.

Montgomery, K. (1991). *Doctors' stories: The narrative structure of medical knowledge.* Princeton: Princeton University Press.

Morris, D.B. (1998). *Illness and culture in the postmodern age.* Berkeley: University of California Press.

Morris, D.B. (2001). Narrative, ethics, and thinking with stories. *Narrative, 9,* 55-77.

Morris, W.E. (2001). David Hume. In Edward Zalta (Ed.), *The Stanford encyclopedia of philosophy.* Retrieved March 1, 2005 from Stanford University's website: http://plato.stanford.edu/archives/spr2001/entries/hume/

The new shorter Oxford English dictionary. (1993). Professionalism (p. 2368). Oxford: Claredon Press.

Nelson, H.L. (Ed.). (1997). *Stories and their limits: Narrative approaches to bioethics.* New York: Routledge.

Novack, D.H., Suchman, A.L., Clark, W., Epstein, R.M., Najberg, E., & Kaplan, M.D. (1997). Calibrating the physician: Personal awareness and effective patient care. *Journal of the American Medical Association, 278,* 502-509.

Pellegrino, E.D. (1985). The virtuous physician and the ethics of medicine. In E.E. Shelp (Ed.), *Virtue and medicine: Exploration in the character of medicine* (Philosophy and Medicine series, 17; pp. 243-55). Dordrecht, Holland: D. Reidel Publishing Company.

Pellegrino, E.D. (1989). Character, virtue and self-interest in the ethics of the professions. *Journal of Contemporary Health Law Policy, 5,* 53-73.

Pellegrino, E.D., & Thomasma, D.C. (1993). *The virtues in medical practice.* New York: Oxford University Press.

Physicians for Human Rights. (2005). *Islamic code of medical ethics.* Retrieved March 1, 2001 from the Physicians for Human Rights website:http://www.phrusa.org/research/methics/methicsoath.html

Pololi, L., Frankel, R.M., Clay, M., & Jobe, A. (2000). One year's experience with a program to facilitate personal and professional development in medical students using reflection groups. *Education for Health, 14*(1), 36-49.

Rothman, D.J. (2000). Medical professionalism—focusing on the real issues. *New England Journal of Medicine, 342,* 1284-1286.

Stephenson, A., Higgs R., & Sugarman, J.(2001). Teaching professional development in medical schools. *The Lancet, 357,* 867-870.

Sulmasy, D.P. (1997). *The healer's calling.* New York: The Paulist Press.

Swick, H.M., Szenas, P., Danoff, D., & Whitcomb, M.E. (1999). Teaching professionalism in undergraduate medical education. *Journal of the American Medical Association, 282,* 830-832.

Wear, D. (1998). On white coats and professional development: The formal and hidden curricula. *Annals of Internal Medicine, 129,* 734-737.

Wear D., & Castellani, B. (2000). The development of professionalism: Curriculum matters. *Academic Medicine, 75,* 602-611.

Veatch, R.M. (1985). Against virtue: A deontological critique of virtue theory in medical ethics. In E.E. Shelp (Ed.), *Virtue and medicine: Exploration in the character of medicine* (Philosophy and Medicine series, 17; pp. 329-45). Dordrecht, Holland: D. Reidel Publishing Company.

Chapter 7

THE ROLE OF ETHICS WITHIN PROFESSIONALISM INQUIRY
Defining Identity and Distinguishing Boundary

Julie M. Aultman
Northeastern Ohio Universities College of Medicine

As a philosopher and medical educator, I have experienced the angst of teaching medical humanities to those students who believe and openly voice that medical humanities courses are "a waste of their time" and are ineffective in teaching them how to be good doctors. While there are a handful of students who do appreciate having courses in the humanities and enter the classroom with open minds and an overall desire to learn as much as they can, my concern rests with those students who enter the classroom with negative attitudes, wrongfully assuming that we are here to tell them how to feel, act, think, and believe in order to be professional—in order to be good doctors.

Upon confronting my disinclined students, I have learned that much of their negativity stems from a learned misinterpretation and misunderstanding of what professionalism is and its relation to ethics, along with the disbelief that moral philosophy, literature, and other courses in the humanities can impact their professional and moral development. I have also learned that even among medical educators who teach courses on professionalism and ethics, these areas of inquiry and application are poorly understood or are ostensibly taught under the assumption that students do not need to know, for example, the theoretical basis for understanding such concepts as "duty" or "altruism," and why these concepts have different implications within professionalism and ethics.

Although a discussion about the importance of humanities in medical education as vehicles for professional growth should not be dismissed given my aforementioned concerns, a related, but more critical topic of discussion is the misinterpretation and misunderstanding of what professionalism is and its relation to ethics, especially medical ethics. As the professionalism movement continues throughout medical education, there lies the danger, as Delese Wear and Mark Kuczewski (2004) write, that "we educators will simply rename what has been called 'medical ethics' as 'professionalism' in the curriculum and consider ourselves done" (p. 4). As a newer breed of ethics continues to emerge in medical education—medical ethics—the boundaries between ethics and professionalism further dissolve, and with it, their loss of identity and effectiveness in medical education.

To avoid this danger, we must develop a better understanding of ethics, or more specifically, medical ethics, and professionalism. Though many of the concepts and values explored within these areas are similar, there are important distinctions in the approaches and goals used to identify and understand these values and the contexts in which they are evaluated. By distinguishing some boundaries between medical ethics and professionalism, we can better determine the role ethics ought to play *within* professionalism inquiry without losing its identity as a related, but separate, field of study and inquiry, while gaining a deeper understanding of what professionalism is and the role it ought to play in medical education. Furthermore, when we are clearer as to the role medical ethics should play within professionalism, we can more fully understand the roles of other critical areas of study, such as sociology or literature.

WHAT IS ETHICS?

Before exploring the role ethics plays within professionalism, it is important to understand what ethics is and some of the difficulties surrounding its classification. To formulate a better understanding of ethics and its role within professionalism inquiry, I describe both general ethics and medical ethics in the following section. There is no one particular way to describe and classify ethics, since there are multiple kinds of thinking within ethics and different contexts in which ethics is understood and used. The way I describe ethics here is to give you, my interdisciplinary readers, an idea of its complexity and its relation to professionalism without departing from my previously addressed aims.

Ethics

Ethics is the philosophical analysis of morality, or the study of not what *is* but what *ought to be*. Ethics critically evaluates the rightness and wrongness of actions and considers how we judge and justify our intentions, motives, and goals as good or bad. Specifically, ethics is the study of moral deliberation, decision-making, and justification; it involves the analysis of behavior and how behavior shapes our character and our relationships with others.

There are three kinds of thinking that relate to morality: descriptive thinking, normative thinking, and meta-ethical thinking. In descriptive thinking, the goal is to describe or explain human nature, i.e., what people are doing and how they are behaving and thinking. The second kind of moral thinking, normative thinking, asks what should be right, good, or obligatory. The final kind of moral thinking, known as meta-ethical thinking, is the logical analysis of moral language. Meta-ethics examines the meaning of ethical terms such as "right," "wrong," "good," and "bad" and related concepts such as responsibility, promise keeping, and duty. If we were to look at, for example, a teenage friendship through the lens of general ethics, we can describe a sixteen year-old girl lying to her friend. This descriptive way of thinking does not provide any evaluative judgments; it only reports an individual's behavior, i.e., lying. From a normative perspective, an ethicist may look at this particular friendship and judge, "the act of lying is *wrong*," or that "the sixteen year-old *should not* lie to her friend." It is from this perspective where we introduce our moral language, using terms like "good," "bad," "wrong," "right," and "should (not)," or "ought (not)," when making a moral judgment. From a meta-ethical perspective, an ethicist may analyze the moral claim that "lying is wrong" by questioning the meaning of "wrong."

In determining which actions are right or wrong or which motives, intentions, and goals are good or bad, moral philosophers have developed ethical theories. Ethical theories interpret our values, guide our moral decisions, and attempt to articulate and justify principles or guidelines, which express standards for making justified decisions, evaluate actions and policies, and make sure our decisions are not based on prejudices or biases. In *Morality and the Professional Life*, Cynthia Brincat and Victoria Wike (2000) illustrate two tasks of such theories: They provide an orientation toward moral situations and resolve conflicts among rules and values (p. 112).

In brief, there are several different ethical theories, and while there are different schemata for organizing them, I found the most useful way to organize these theories is to determine whether they focus on actions or kinds of action or on persons, including their motives and traits of character (Frankena, 1973, p. 9). The principle-based theories, or theories that generate guidelines to direct our actions, include goal-based, duty-based, and rights-based theories, which focus on how a person ought to act. The theories without principles, including virtue theory, ethics of care, and narrative, focus on the status of that person, i.e., what characterizes and differentiates this person from others, including her character, the nature of her relationships with others, and her life story.

Though each ethical theory is useful, no one theory in particular can interpret all of our moral values, guide all of our moral decisions, or resolve all of our moral dilemmas. However, by carefully weighing each theory, along with individual beliefs and non-philosophical theories, which may be culturally, spiritually, or socially based for each individual, we can begin to identify, deliberate, and resolve ethical conflict, while reflecting upon the moral judgments we make. Essentially, ethics is a systematic approach for understanding ourselves as persons and how we make moral decisions; it is a critical and reflective examination of how we ought to live in relation to others.

Medical Ethics

Stemming from the Hippocratic tradition, medical ethics was a way physicians could govern their own conduct. It wasn't until the 1970s that medical ethics (or "bioethics" as it is sometimes referred) began to be more representative of moral philosophy, with theories and principles outside of Hippocratic medical ethics. As medical ethics progressed, physicians also became more reliant on others outside the field of medicine (such as philosophers and theologians) to provide a critical, unbiased, and coherent approach for guiding beliefs and actions and for resolving moral conflict.

Today medical ethics addresses a variety of normative and meta-ethical concepts and issues, along with ideas stemming from the philosophy of medicine that are not necessarily professional matters, such as concepts of "disease," "normalcy," and so on. Medical ethics involves similar methods of moral reasoning and inquiry as general ethics, though these methods are specifically directed toward issues and problems within medicine.

In looking at the previous case of the sixteen year-old girl who lies to her friend, medical ethicists would not be concerned with this particular case *per se*, since lying to one's friend is not an ethical problem relevant to medicine. However, medical ethicists would be concerned with physicians lying to their patients. Similar to general ethics, descriptions and judgments are made (e.g., lying is wrong), and similar questions may be asked, (e.g., "Is lying *always* morally wrong?"). Still, cases outside of medicine can be very useful to the medical ethicist; cases such as the lying teenager can be used for comparison, i.e., when physicians think about lying to their patient to determine whether similar moral judgments are made and why.

Philosophers and educators, such as Brincat and Wike (2000), view medical ethics as a type of professional ethics. Though medical ethics could very well be viewed as a type of professional ethics, it should be clearly noted that many of the questions of medical ethics do not focus solely on the profession of medicine, or even doctors for that matter. Furthermore, the boundaries between general ethics and medical ethics are not always clear, and thus, complicate not only how we understand medical ethics but also how we understand its role within professionalism inquiry.

One of the forerunners of professional ethics, Alan Goldman (1980), critically looks at the role of ethics in one's professional life and questions whether particular ethical guidelines and norms are required to guide the conduct and render the character of the professional or whether traditional principles should apply. In his examination of Goldman's work, John Lawrence (1999) writes, "He sees a professional role as strongly differentiated if it requires unique principles, or if it requires its norms to be weighted more heavily than they would be against other principles in other contexts. In this case the professional must elevate certain values or goals, those central to his or her profession, such as health, or legal autonomy of clients, to the status of overriding considerations" (p. 26).

For purposes of distinguishing *some* of the differences between general ethics and medical ethics and for explaining what role medical ethics has within professionalism, I maintain that medical ethics is a type of professional ethics, though it encompasses much more than the moral evaluation and regulation of the professions (a trap that educators often fall into when teaching professional ethics). Also, medical ethics is an area of study that is and should be distinct from professionalism, since it addresses ethical issues and concepts (as well as concepts from the philosophy of medicine, metaphysics and epistemology) that are of little concern for those who study, teach, and strive for professionalism.

In explaining some of the differences between general ethics and medical ethics, Brincat and Wike (2000) suggest the primary difference is the audiences at which general ethics and medical ethics are aimed. While general ethics aims to provide a moral framework for every individual within the moral community who "share in the moral benefits and obligations in which all of humanity participates," medical ethics as a type of professional ethics focuses only on those individuals who are members of the [medical] profession (Brincat & Wike, 2000, p. 58).

Other differences between general ethics and medical ethics include the topics and concepts identified and discussed. Brincat and Wike (2000) write, "The topics of promise keeping, confidentiality, and fair hiring practices are just as important to general ethics as they are to professional ethics. But the importance of these issues to general ethics is the importance that stems from their reliance on general ethical commitments that we all share" (Brincat & Wike, 2000, p. 58).

As the medical profession has become more complex with the advancement of technology, along with recognition of community and global interests and needs, there has been a greater need for medical ethics to guide individuals to identify, deliberate, resolve, and reflect upon complicated moral dilemmas, and to develop codes and policies to guide future actions and commitments within the medical profession. Medical ethics can be an important element within professionalism inquiry, since it not only forces us to examine practical issues and dilemmas among a wider community audience, but also guides us in developing important analytical, critical thinking, and imaginative skills as traditional ethical methods of moral reasoning are employed. The role of medical ethics within professionalism inquiry, then, will be the topic of discussion within the next few sections.

WHAT IS PROFESSIONALISM?

At the end of her fourth and final year at medical school, a student whom I will refer to as "Katie," completed an independent research project on professionalism and moral development in medical education. In putting this project together, I asked Katie to reflect upon the past four years, identifying those experiences and relationships that contributed to her understanding of professionalism and how this understanding has shaped the way she views herself as a person. The result of her independent study was a remarkable, honest perspective on what she understood professionalism to be, how and why many topics of professionalism are generally devalued by medical students, along with some of the major challenges medical educators face in teaching professionalism.

What initially struck me in Katie's portrayal of medical school and how professionalism is introduced and taught was the vast amount of definitions and rule-based codes of professionalism she was exposed to throughout her four years, all of which had little meaning to her and her peers. While Katie explained that professionalism "incorporates characteristics such as altruism, accountability and responsibility, respect, honor, leadership, skill and excellence, caring, compassion, and communication," she admitted having never been overtly taught what these characteristics or attributes mean or how to resolve ethical, social, and legal dilemmas when a conflict among them may develop in the clinical setting. Katie experienced a deliberate and unreflective "push for professionalism," beginning with the traditional White Coat Ceremony and continuing throughout her education with mandatory lectures in the behavioral sciences and various humanities courses, where she, along with her peers, were told how to feel, think, and act in order to develop "good" communication and interpersonal skills with their patients and colleagues.

Though Katie believes these courses that "push for professionalism" are a good starting place, she believes "there is always room for improvement," beginning with discussions about students' understanding of professionalism and those attributes that seem to be relevant to their personal and professional growth. How she began to understand the meaning of professionalism and its importance within medical education and practice was not through traditional rituals or exercises and lectures on how to talk to your patient, but through critical reflection of her feelings and experiences, and the feelings and experiences of others. This ability to critically reflect, developed over the course of her four years at medical school, and was shaped by both positive and negative influences. In describing these positive and negative influences Katie, citing from Hilton (2004), writes:

> Professionalism is acquired over many years through a combination of both positive and negative influences in a medical student's life. Positive influences over this time include a supportive learning environment, constructive role models, social involvement, and experiences with assessments that promote reflective learning within and outside of the hospital . . . compared to negative effects such as unhelpful teaching, negative role models, unsupportive work conditions, and pressure of overwork. In the end, the degree of professionalism becomes dependent upon the interaction between the positive and negative influences.

To better understand how other medical students understand professionalism, Katie asked many of her peers to explain what professionalism meant to them. Admittedly, her peers had as much difficulty as Katie in coming up with an adequate working definition of professionalism. She explained that no two persons' answers were the same, and thus turned to "the experts" to find the meaning of professionalism.

The American Board of Internal Medicine (ABIM), for example, defines professionalism in the following way: "Professionalism in medicine requires the physician to serve the interests of the patient above his or her self-interest. Professionalism *aspires* to altruism, accountability, excellence, duty, service, honor, integrity and respect for others" (p. 5). Related to this definition are seven issues that challenge or diminish the previously identified elements of professionalism: abuse of power, arrogance, greed, misrepresentation, impairment, lack of conscientiousness, and conflict of interest. Furthermore, the ABIM suggests three elements, or commitments, of professionalism required of candidates seeking certification or re-certification. These commitments, outlined in their 1999 publication, *Project Professionalism*, include "a commitment to the highest standards of excellence in the practice of medicine and in the generation and dissemination of knowledge, a commitment to sustain the interests and welfare of patients, and a commitment to be responsive to the health needs of society" (p. 5).

Though the ABIM does report those important attributes and commitments that health care professionals should strive for in their practice of medicine, the ABIM, as with several other groups, fails to describe what, for example, is the meaning of "excellence," how to obtain it, measure it, and maintain it, and its relation to being a "good" professional. Nevertheless, "excellence" is used in this report as both a virtue and a description of those standards to which one ought to be committed; it "entails a conscientious effort to exceed ordinary expectations and to make a commitment to life-long learning" (p. 6). For the medical student or resident who is struggling to understand the meaning of excellence, she may, for example, "exceed ordinary expectations" by taking a greater patient load. But the motivation behind taking a greater patient load may be based on self-interest or convenience. And is taking a greater patient load really an act of excellence? How do we know when our actions or when a person's character resembles those attributes defined in the ABIM?

Thomas Inui, author of an AAMC publication *A Flag in the Wind: Educating for Professionalism in Medicine* (2003), recognizes a variety of definitions (or "taxonomies of domains") that characterize what professionalism is and what physicians should aspire to embody or exemplify through actions, attitudes, and values, including altruism, honor, and integrity, caring, compassion, respect, responsibility, accountability, excellence and scholarship, and leadership. Inui continues:

> These various descriptions are so similar because when we examine the field of medicine as a *profession*, a field of work in which the workers must be implicitly trustworthy, we end by realizing and asserting that they must pursue their work as *a virtuous activity, a moral understanding*. All explications of professionalism then devolve into

descriptions of the general qualities of a virtuous person, one who works in the field of medicine, and how such a virtuous person would act. (p. 14)

Although Inui and others understand that professionalism encompasses important qualities a person working in the profession of medicine ought to possess, the problem with approaching professionalism in this manner, i.e., listing attributes that individuals should possess, is that there is no guidance for acquiring these attributes or virtues. If a physician is and should be accountable to self, patients, society, and the profession, how will she make a choice when, for example, accountability to patients conflicts with accountability to legal standards? Katie experienced how difficult it was to find a clear and consistent explanation of professionalism and what means to be professional and thus, realizes how necessary it is, as Wear and Kuczewski recommend, to pause and take stock in what has been said, who has been speaking, and for whom the professionalism discourse is intended (Wear & Kuczewski, 2004, p. 8). At the end of her project, Katie explained how she really never sat down to think about issues of professionalism and its relationship to medical ethics beyond those attributes to which she was told to aspire.

Understanding professionalism, then, can be a difficult task. The educational challenge of such inquiry is to create an open discursive forum to understand more fully the values and beliefs that circulate between and around doctors, patients, and other health care professionals; the medical institutions in which they work and the corporate entities influencing that work; and the local, national, and global communities. Professionalism inquiry, then, is an integrative approach or method for developing students' reflective awareness of those values and beliefs. Such inquiry requires medical educators to create and maintain a discourse through which students can identify and examine specific elements of professionalism, including the virtues or attributes that characterize the professional; regulations and policies that guide the profession; and the needs, goals, and ideals of the patients and communities they serve.

To further understand the nature of professionalism, I elaborate next on medical ethics, one of the elements within professionalism inquiry, to show how it, among other areas of study, provides the foundations of professionalism through which tradition, experience, skill, and character contribute to the personal and professional development of individuals and to the overall culture of the medical profession.

THE RELATIONSHIP BETWEEN MEDICAL ETHICS AND PROFESSIONALISM INQUIRY

In this section I address two important questions: What role should medical ethics play in professionalism? What may be some of the difficulties in understanding this role?

Frederic Hafferty (2000) illustrates how medical ethics has been an integral part of professionalism, in general, by providing not only a theoretical base from which certain attributes or virtues can be better explained and understood, but also the critical reasoning tools required to identify moral issues, resolve dilemmas and conflicts among professional attributes, and reflect upon moral decisions once they are made and the effects these decisions may have on others within and external to the medical community. Yet John Kultgen (1988) points out a well-known fact about professionals, which I have witnessed in teaching medical students: They are impatient with the fretted questions of medical ethics, feeling as though they have "been raised in good homes and are God-fearing, church going men [*sic*]." This is a particular challenge to medical educators to persuade those who are impatient with these "fretted questions of ethics" to be more reflective of their personal values, especially in relation to their professional lives.

My fourth year medical student, Katie, has confirmed this reality, indicating that she, like many of her peers, imagined that all the ethics she needed came from her family life and experiences prior to medical school. Nevertheless, Katie reported, "Although students bring to medical school a fairly well established value system, the potential for moral growth through the next four years is substantial." Little did she realize the ethical complexities surrounding both her professional and personal life that would challenge her beliefs, judgments, and behavior. However, unlike some professionals who do not understand the importance of ethical inquiry and training and "take personal offense at criticisms of their professional conduct," Katie has begun to understand how the questions of medical ethics are useful for working through difficult issues and situations within her personal and professional life.

Similar to what Katie expresses is Charles Culver's (1985) understanding of the role of medical ethics in "making good doctors." He argues that "the basic moral character of medical students has been formed by the time they enter medical school. A medical ethics curriculum is designed not to improve the moral character of future physicians, but to provide those of sound moral character with the intellectual tools and interactional skills to give that moral character its best behavioral expression"(p. 238).

Furthermore, medical ethics guides the professional to consider the values held by her patients and others. By considering those values, the medical student can begin to understand who the patient is, what it is like to be the patient, and follow a professional course of action that reflects a careful, respectful consideration of the patient's values without imposing personal values on him or her. However, for students to acquire important skills and tools to work through difficult issues, identify personal and professional values and beliefs, and understand the values and beliefs of others, their teachers must also not be impatient with "fretted questions of ethics." When medical educators do not have the skills or expertise in ethics, but insist on inserting the ubiquitous "case discussion" at every turn because "that is what professionalism is about," students receive a limited ethics education outside of philosophy. Arguably, medical ethics is not ethics without foundations in philosophy. Medical ethics outside philosophy is a mess of entangled disciplines, approaching contentious issues or topics from different perspectives with no independent, theoretical ground to support these perspectives or the ideas, questions, and answers that may arise from them.

Ioanna Kucuradi (1999) reveals how there has been a renaissance of ethics outside philosophy—an "outburst of various professional ethics" (p. 2). While there can be an ethics outside of philosophy, an ethics *based* on the guiding principles of philosophical ethics, this ethics is limited and is not a good approach for regulating a profession or serving a community; it does not allow health care professionals and others to develop important practical skills such as critical thinking, which enables them to recognize, reason, resolve, and reflect on difficult (moral, social, legal, personal, and so forth) conflicts.

Furthermore, as medical ethics has become more popular in medical education, I have witnessed "ethics" educators and administrators, i.e., those with little or no training in ethics as a philosophical area of study, present case studies to students and colleagues with the expectation that ethical issues and dilemmas can be resolved through lengthy and collective discussions about the case. Though the presentation of cases can be an important step in getting students and others to think about difficult issues, the problem lies in how students are guided in their thinking. What typically occurs when an "ethicist" leads a case discussion, is the application of ethical rules and principles, which are expected to help students "automatically" resolve the case, i.e., which ever rule or principle *appears* to fit the best, is the one which will guide the students' actions or beliefs. However, as a result, students tend to use ethical theories and principles in a cookbook fashion, applying them to any issue or situation without understanding their history, complexity, and significance, and often confuse ethics with law, religion, or anthropological/sociological theory, or worse yet, their unfounded opinions.

What *should* happen is a discussion about all the elements of the case (including those elements which may be missing), and not just the obvious ethical dilemmas the presenter wants others to see, as well as an explanation as to how and why certain ethical theories and principles may be useful in guiding particular actions and/or beliefs. Most students have not yet developed the skills needed to identify, deliberate, resolve, and reflect upon the issues and dilemmas contained in a given ethics case. By lacking these important skills (such as critical thinking), students rely on what they know, including biases and prejudices they perceive as "normal" or "morally appropriate," without considering other values and beliefs that may guide them toward a better resolution of a case or reaffirm their own beliefs and values.

In addition, "ethics" educators and administrators tend to present cases that can and have been resolved; they rarely, if ever, present hypothetical or fictional cases where students learn to use their imaginations in thinking about possible methods (and outcomes) for identifying and resolving ethical dilemmas. By presenting cases that can and have been resolved, educators and administrators are sending the message to students that ethical and moral reasoning is easy, and the sole purpose of the exercise is to find an answer or make a resolution.

Moreover, we should not assume that just because some medical educators' areas of expertise fit under the rubric of professionalism, they are also experts in medical ethics. Now, I am not suggesting that educators should not teach or do research outside of their areas of expertise, or that faculty development in medical ethics is an unattainable goal in medical education. What I *am* suggesting is that we should support educators and what they bring to students' moral and professional development by preserving and respecting their areas of expertise. Teaching professionalism does not mean teaching a single course "on professionalism" that covers a list of virtues or principles relevant to the practice of medicine. Teaching professionalism means teaching important concepts, theories, values, issues, and dilemmas, arising from a variety of deeply rooted academic disciplines and areas of study (e.g., sociology), which provide students with *personal* and *professional* skills, values, and behaviors important for establishing themselves as health care professionals *and* members of their communities who have rich and meaningful personal lives as well.

To preserve the identity of medical ethics, and not to confuse medical ethics with professionalism, we need to distinguish boundaries while identifying a possible overlap between the two, i.e., the role medical ethics plays within professionalism inquiry.

Approaches in medical ethics useful for professionalism inquiry

Examining the role of medical ethics within professionalism inquiry entails determining which approaches or types of moral reasoning should be included. There are several approaches for moral reasoning that are particularly useful for building professionals' critical thinking, communication and imaginative skills and for developing professional codes and policies, among other activities within a professionalism curriculum. The approaches include principlism, casuistry, and virtue theory.

Principlism, an action-based approach, has been quite influential, since it focuses not on abstract moral theory but on common moral experience through a set of middle-level norms or principles. Four primary principles identified by Tom Beauchamp and James Childress in the 1970s—autonomy, beneficence, non-maleficence, and justice—are consistent with moral theory, but articulate particular moral duties in a simpler way, thus making moral reasoning more accessible to non-theorists. Reasoning through moral issues and conflicts occurs when the principles are weighed and balanced against one another, often resulting in a type of ranking where one or more principles have priority over the others in a given situation.

For example, when a patient in a persistent vegetative state refuses a feeding tube (as she stated in the form of a living will prior to her current medical status), the physician may weigh the principle of non-maleficence, which directs the physician to "do no harm," against the principle of autonomy, which directs the physician to respect the wishes of the patient. However, in this case, the principles may conflict with each other, especially if the physician interprets the removal of the feeding tube as an act of harm. Thus, there can be serious problems with this approach.

First, principlism merely states what the moral duties are and how they should be ranked in a particular situation; it does not explain what these principles actually mean or how competing principles settle moral conflicts. In other words, because principlism lacks foundational theory, decision making and conflict resolution appear subjective and action is not adequately determined.

Second, principlism is what is known as a "top-down" way of thinking where you begin with the principles and work your way down to specific cases and situations. Because of this linear way of thinking, principles tend to be "applied" mechanically to situations and often times by novices who believe they have become experts in medical ethics "because they can chant the mantra" (Childress, 2001, p. 69). However, not all principle-based approaches are as deductivistic or mechanical as principlism.

Another approach is situation-based. One example of a situation-based approach that professionalism borrows is casuistry. Casuistry, or case-based reasoning, is when specific cases are used to inform moral principles. That is, instead of starting out with a set of principles, the casuist begins with a particular case and "branches out to analogous cases of greater complexity and difficulty . . . responding to the particularities of different settings, treatments, and categories" (Steinbock, Arras, & London, 2003, p. 39). Casuists believe that our examination of cases, rather than abstract theories and principles, bring us closer to moral certitude. Unlike "top down" or "theory driven" methods, casuistry is a type of "bottom-up" thinking, i.e., we begin with a case and work our way up to the development of abstract moral rules or principles. Casuistry is an attractive approach for inclusion within professionalism, since "it is a method of thinking especially well-suited to busy physicians and nurses whose clinical outlook is already thoroughly case-oriented and who have neither the time nor the inclination to bother with too much theory" (Arras, 2001, p. 110).

However, similar to principlism, there are a number of criticisms surrounding this approach for moral reasoning. In brief, casuistry is insufficiently critical. Synopsizing what critics of casuistry have said, John Arras (2001) writes, "A common objection to casuistical approaches is that, precisely because they work from the 'bottom up'—because they begin already immersed in current intuitions, convictions, and practices – they are unable to provide a critical standpoint from which those very practices might by judged" (p. 112).

Some critics believe that because casuistry requires one to have a vast amount of knowledge about paradigms, it is difficult for individuals to draw parallels from these pure cases to real life situations, or as Arras explains, "Reasoning by analogy is too indeterminate" (p. 112). Casuistry has also been criticized as specious; it is only most effective when collective discussion and reasoning occurs.

A third type of approach for moral reasoning, virtue theory, is a character-based approach grounded in traditional moral theory. It is not uncommon for professionals, educators, and others to assume that the type of ethical theory that should be part of professionalism is virtue theory because most, if not all, definitions and descriptions of professionalism involve a set of virtues or attributes to which the professional should aspire. Though virtue medical ethics can be an integral part of professionalism, it should not be the only ethical theory in which students, professionals, and others utilize. Because virtue ethics only focuses on the character of the professional, it fails to *guide* her choices and actions. Another common argument against virtue ethics is when virtues conflict, there is no way for the professional to rank or determine which values should take precedent over other values.

What is required for moral reasoning, deliberation, decision-making, and reflecting—and I would argue, professionalism inquiry—is the careful consideration and weighing of various ethical theories and principles; no one particular theory or principle can resolve a moral dilemma or ethical controversy, and no one individual can make moral judgments without the consideration of others.

As I see it, the best ethical approach that meets the unique demands of professionalism inquiry is an approach that draws upon multiple approaches such as principlism, casuistry, and virtue ethics. Furthermore, to achieve critical morality, we must not only consider moral theories, principles, and cases, but also our background beliefs and theories about the world, such as those examined in other disciplines such as anthropology or history, bringing them into a coherent framework through which moral deliberation, decision-making, and reflection can take place. The type of moral reasoning that directs our attention to the needs of others and helps us recognize social and community roles is what is required within the rubric of professionalism, especially since it is able to bring other areas of study into the framework for a better understanding of situations, persons, relationships, motivations, and so forth.

Indeed, the recognition of social and community roles within medical ethics and professionalism inquiry has changed the view that professionalism is just about doctors and the guidelines and codes that guide their practices. Professionalism as a mode of inquiry must also incorporate various sociological, cultural, spiritual, and political elements so that students and others can create a systematic framework for understanding and organizing the nature of their profession, what it means to be a doctor, and what both patient and societal needs can and should be met. While medical ethics is an important element within this professional inquiry, it should not dominate or replace these other disciplinary and personal elements that contribute to professional development in medicine. What professionalism should take from medical ethics are the skills acquired through philosophical, ethical inquiry and reasoning. However, medical ethics should be understood and taught as a distinguishable area of study through which students can gain greater insight into some of the ethical issues and dilemmas of our day that may have little direct ties to professionalism inquiry.

WHERE TO FROM HERE? A PROFESSIONALISM CURRICULUM

As Audiey Kao (2004) suggests, the professionalism movement "might be employed by some as a way of 'advertising' humanistic training to skeptical students and faculty" who have not taken ethics education seriously (p. 49). To avoid the marginalization of professionalism education, his solution is to create a formal curriculum in professionalism, design faculty development programs, and give priority to teaching as a core mission.

In designing a formal curriculum and placing greater focus on teaching, it is imperative for medical educators to teach students not only how to care for their patients but to value themselves in relation to their patients. That is, before students can understand and actually experience empathy, compassion, integrity, and all the so-called virtues of being a doctor, they need to learn about themselves (i.e., identifying their personal values and beliefs, including how they obtained them and whether they are willing to change them in light of new experiences or information) before identifying, judging, and comparing their patients' values and beliefs with their own and the standards of the profession. By gaining further knowledge about themselves, students begin to confront personal biases and prejudices, and hopefully begin the lifelong process of unlearning them.

A curriculum in professionalism should be an integral part of the overall medical school experience and should be well-respected among students and faculty alike. However, in order for this curriculum to be successful, students, clinical and non-clinical faculty, and administrative personnel of any given medical school need to be aware of the importance of professionalism beyond its superficial definitions and categories of virtues. One possible approach for raising awareness is to involve students, faculty, and administrative personnel in a collective activity, where professionalism is understood through community participation. Whether a problem in professionalism is discussed, e.g., whistle blowing, or general forums or "conferences" are created for individuals to openly speak of issues and concerns involving the educational environment, patient care, collegiality, and so on, awareness can begin by collectively discussing issues of professionalism.

However, these methods for raising awareness can be unsuccessful if we are not careful, especially if faculty and administrative personnel assume paternalistic roles and tell students how to think, believe, act, and feel in order to be professional. Faculty and administrators must remember they too are confronted with professional issues and dilemmas, and not just those who are or will be engaged in clinical practice. Students can only understand respect, honesty, and humility if their role models treat them with respect and are honest and humble when discussing professionalism.

Although my expertise is in ethics, as a medical educator I have recognized a need for a curriculum in professionalism where medical ethics and philosophy of medicine are just a few areas of study among many. The professionalism curriculum should also include course work in literature, art, sociology and public health, religious studies, medical anthropology, the history of science and medicine, law, and political theory. These courses should be more advanced than those taken throughout students' undergraduate education and should focus on issues and problems relevant to becoming a doctor; to patients and their families; to educational, clinical, and community environments, including how to interact and work with residents, nurses, and other clinical and non-clinical individuals, the hospital culture, professional and personal obligations and responsibilities; plus those issues that affect all persons such as gender, race, ethnicity, sexual identity, and so on. This coursework should begin at the start of medical school and continue throughout medical education.

Students should also be given a variety of assignments not limited to the specific content of their humanities courses. Their assignments should integrate their course content along with their perspectives and experiences on the subject matter as it relates to their personal and professional lives. They should be given a variety of writing assignments such as personal, reflective essays and patient narratives based on real patient interviews and ethical case studies. Students should also be exposed to unfamiliar persons, places, and belief systems through fictional and non-fictional short stories, novels, religious doctrines, and art. Each of these assignments should be designed to enhance students' communication, critical and creative thinking skills, and to develop their abilities to self-reflect and identify what others may be feeling or experiencing when they are ill. In fact, until students begin to recognize their own prejudices and biases and develop the skills they need to identify, reason, and reflect upon personal issues and dilemmas, they will not be able to grasp the virtues to which they are expected to aspire, such as empathy and compassion.

To reiterate, in gaining a better understanding of medical professionalism and how it ought to be taught, refined, and reflected upon, we must begin by identifying the theoretical groundwork of philosophy (and other areas of study) from which professional concepts, problems, rules and principles, objectives, and so forth develop. What we see throughout medical education are directives and statements indicating how a person ought to be or act in order to be professional and how an institution should operate in order to foster professionalism. What we do *not* see are the reasons and meanings behind these directives and statements, e.g., why a person should act compassionately, or what compassion means and its significance in the medical profession. Definitions, guidelines, and objectives are not enough for understanding professionalism or for becoming a professional.

As I argued above, the role of medical ethics within professionalism does not represent all the concepts, methods or theories of medical ethics, just as medical ethics does not represent all that general ethics has to offer. Thus, we must establish boundaries between the two by gaining a deeper, clearer, and consistent understanding of what professionalism is (and should be) and what medical ethics is (and should be). In addition, when we conceptualize medical professionalism, our efforts will be enhanced when we consider the medical, ethical/moral, psychological, sociological, literary, cultural, religious, political, and legal areas of inquiry that inform doctoring, the experience of illness, and our overall understanding of the values intrinsic to the medical profession, of what it means to be a professional, and of the communities the professional interacts with and serves.

REFERENCES

American Board of Internal Medicine (1999). *Project professionalism.* Philadelphia: ABIM Communications.

Arras, J. (2001). A case approach. In H. Kuhse & P. Singer (Eds.), *A companion to bioethics* (pp. 106-114). Malden, MA: Blackwell Publishers.

Brincat, C., & Wike, V. (2000). *Morality and the professional life: Values at work.* New Jersey: Prentice Hall.

Childress, J. F. (2001). A principle-based approach. In H. Kuhse & P. Singer (Eds.), *A companion to bioethics* (pp. 61-71). Malden, MA: Blackwell Publishers.

Culver, C.M. (1985). Basic curricular goals in medical ethics. *New England Journal of Medicine, 312*(4), 253.

Frankena, W.K. (1973). *Ethics*. New Jersey: Prentice-Hall.

Goldman, A.H. (1980). *The moral foundations of professional ethics*. New Jersey: Rowman & Littlefield Publishers.

Hafferty, F. (2000). In search of a lost cord: Professionalism and medical education's hidden curriculum. In D. Wear & J. Bickel (Eds.), *Educating for professionalism: Creating a culture of humanism in medical education* (pp. 11-34). Iowa City: University of Iowa Press.

Hilton, S. (2004). The basics of clinical practice. Medical professionalism: How can we encourage it in our students? *The Clinical Teacher, 1*, 69. Retrieved June 14, 2005 from the website: http://www.blackwell-synergy.com/links/doi/10.1111/j.1743-498x.2004.000032.x/full/

Inui, T.S. (2003). *A flag in the wind: Educating for professionalism in medicine*. Washington, DC: Association of American Medical Colleges.

Kao, A. (2004). Pausing for professionalism. *The American Journal of Bioethics, 4*(2), 49-50.

Kuçuradi, I. (Ed.). (1999). *Ethics of the professions: Medicine, business, media, law* (Studies in economic ethics and philosophy). Berlin, Germany: Springer-Verlag.

Kultgen, J. (1988). *Ethics and professionalism*. Philadelphia: University of Pennsylvania Press.

Lawrence, J. (1999). *Argument for action: Ethics and professional conduct*. Brookfield, VT: Ashgate.

Steinbock, B., Arras, J.D., & London, A.J. (2003). *Ethical issues in modern medicine* (6th edition). Boston: McGraw-Hill.

Wear, D., & Kuczewski, M. (2004). The professionalism movement: Can we pause? *The American Journal of Bioethics, 4*(2), 1-10.

Chapter 8

MEDICAL PROFESSIONALS AND THE DISCOURSE OF PROFESSIONALISM
Teaching Implications

Bradley Lewis
New York University

In the Spring 2004 issue of *The American Journal of Bioethics* (*AJOB*), Delese Wear and Mark Kuczewski initiated a discourse analysis of the professionalism movement in medical education. Wear and Kuczewski's article, "The Professionalism Movement: Can We Pause?," expressed concern that recent medical professionalism pedagogy, ostensibly designed to create compassionate, dutiful, and sensitive physicians, may suffer from a number of serious problems. In this paper, I discuss one such problem: the relationship between the professionalism movement and issues of social context and social justice. I conclude with specific pedagogical and curricular recommendations for the professional development of physicians in training.

Like Wear and Kuczewski I use a discursive approach. Their *AJOB* article was followed by a series of responses and critiques that generated a rich array of perspectives on medical professionalism. Together, the article and its responses provide an ideal opportunity for further discourse analysis. My discursive study of the article and its responses reveals key tensions within the contemporary discourse of professionalism, which create significant incommensurabilities among participants in the discourse. I argue that fine tuning the discourse and being aware of the tensions and incommensurabilities can allow teachers and students of medicine to revitalize the professionalism movement.

WHAT IS DISCOURSE?

But, first, what is discourse analysis? Most of the respondents to the *AJOB* article show little understanding of the specialized meaning of the term in contemporary humanities and social theory. Most skip quickly over Wear and Kuczewski's call for discourse analysis and move directly into their own situated point of view regarding the professionalism movement. Many cite empirical studies of professionalism outcome data or call for more empirical studies of this kind. They imply that empiricism somehow sidesteps discourse and achieves a non-discursive view of truth. This limited familiarity with discourse among medical educators represents the continued cultural gap between the two sides of campus, between humanities and the medical sciences. The concepts of discourse and discursive practices are at the heart of contemporary humanities and social theory, yet they are hardly understood at all in medicine and the biosciences.

The main exception in the *AJOB* issue to this limited familiarity with discourse comes from two respondents from the University of Washington School of Nursing. Jamie Shirley and Stephen Padgett—also contributors to this volume—explain that discourse in contemporary humanities and social theory refers to a socially constructed selection of linguistic signifiers used to understand and perceive the world. These linguistic signifiers organize the interests, values, and priorities of the community that develops them. They also organize the social practices and institutions of the community. As a result, discursive languages "are constitutive of a way of being in the world . . . a form of life. Language is what we do, not merely how we talk about what we do" (Shirley & Padgett, 2004, p. 36).

Discursive forms of life create common sense for its members. The feelings of inevitability, of solidity, and of stability that discourse creates come largely from the experience of being embedded within a given discursive community. However, discursive theory does not imply anything-goes relativity, or that the "real" world plays no role in how communities select their prevailing discourses. Instead, discursive theory stands on the shoulders of postmodern philosophy to move beyond the modernist trap of *either* objectivism *or* relativism. Postmodern philosophy argues *both* that there is a real world *and* that the real world is sufficiently complex to support multiple social constructions that can meaningfully and practically organize it (Lewis, in press).

Discursive theory and postmodern philosophy help make modernist discourses, like contemporary medicine and or the professionalism movement, visible as only one possible "way-of-life" with a specific set of priorities, rituals, institutions, norms, and expectations. Sociologist Zygmunt

Bauman (1990) eloquently captures this sentiment in his discussion of postmodern theory:

> Postmodernity is modernity coming of age: modernity looking at itself at a distance rather than from the inside, making a full inventory of its gains and its losses, psychoanalyzing itself, discovering the intentions it never before spelled out, finding them mutually canceling and incongruous. Postmodernity is modernity coming to terms with its own impossibility; a self-monitoring modernity, one that consciously discards what it was unconsciously doing. (p. 272)

Bauman's version of postmodernism, particularly his anti-utopian emphasis on trade-offs, tough choices, and irreducible conflicts, captures the essence of discourse analysis. Like postmodern theory, discourse analysis is a self-monitoring practice. It does not see evolving discourse as natural, inevitable, or on a path of purified progress, but rather views it as a human practice, and, like other human practices, open to all manner of human limitations.

Bauman's reference to psychoanalysis also provides an important link to understanding the actual method of discourse analysis. Both psychoanalysts and discourse analysts make interpretations not merely to understand phenomena but also to make things better. Freud's psychoanalysis draws attention to patients' prevailing patterns of thought and emotion through interpreting unfiltered free associations. He draws attention particularly to conflicted areas of thought and emotion and to the "unspeakable" aspects of the patient's life (Groth, 1982). The point of such an interpretive practice is not understanding alone. Through interpretations that allow the conflicts and the unspeakable to emerge, the patient is able face what is often most unfaceable about him- or herself, using such insights to make changes for the better. Discourse analysts, in a similar vein, tease out the patterns and conflicts within discursive communities, articulating unspoken dimensions of discursive structures. And like psychoanalysts, they do this so that discursive communities can make changes for the better in their discursive practices.

ANALYZING THE DISCURSIVE CONFLICTS IN MEDICAL PROFESSIONALISM

If we apply this kind of discourse analysis to Wear and Kuczewski's *AJOB* article and the many responses it received, key moments of tension and conflict between the authors emerge. These conflicts result in broad incommensurability among the commentators that leaves them talking past each other regarding two main concerns: First, what does social justice have to do with medical care? Second, what is the role of democracy in medical knowledge making?

Behind both of these incommensurabilities lies a fundamental difference of mindset between discursive members. Some respondents approach medicine through what C. Wright Mills (1959) once termed a "sociological imagination," and some do not. This makes a tremendous difference because whether one works with a sociological imagination or not alters radically one's perception of medicine and professionalism. For Mills, the sociological imagination makes the connection between personal and public issues of a social structure, enabling "its possessor to understand the larger historical scene in terms of its meaning for the inner life and external career of a variety of individuals" (Mills, 1959, p. 5). Within a sociological imagination the personal and the public are very much intertwined: public structures organize private individuals and private individuals organize public structures. Together they become the institutions of a historical society as a whole.

Mill's concept of a sociological imagination helps make sense of the first incommensurability among the *AJOB* responders around the question of social justice and health care. Most of the respondents, working without an active sociological imagination, find the role of social justice in health care vague and obscure. For those working with a sociological imagination, however, the relation between social justice and health care becomes paramount, almost to the point of obscuring all other concerns. Sociologist Irving Zola most eloquently described how the sociological imagination applies to health care. He called it "focusing upstream":

> [A physician once said], sometimes it feels like this. There I am standing by the shore of a swiftly flowing river and I hear the cry of a drowning man. So I jump into the river, put my arms around him, pull him to the shore and apply artificial respiration. Just when he begins to breath, there is another cry for help. So I jump into the river, reach him, pull him to shore, apply artificial respiration, and then just as he begins to breathe, another cry for help. So back in the river again, reaching pulling, applying, breathing and then another yell. Again and again, without end, goes the sequence. You know, I am so busy jumping in, pulling them to shore, applying artificial respiration, that I have no time to see who the hell is upstream pushing them all in. (cited in McKinlay, 2001, p. 516)

Thus, for those working within a sociological imagination, Zola's image of "focusing upstream" vividly concentrates the mind on the social determinants of individual health care problems.

But focusing upstream reveals a painful and, for many, a seemingly unacceptable insight for contemporary medicine. Put most starkly, the unacceptable insight that comes from looking upstream is that the priorities of the dominant forms of "institutional medicine" both *neglect* and *abuse* patients.[1] Clearly, "neglect" and "abuse" are strong terms, even stronger than those used by respondents in the *AJOB* issue who work within a sociological imagination. But if one is going to foreground the tensions surrounding medical professionalism, no other terms sufficiently convey the extent of the problems institutional medicine faces when we look upstream.

Starting with *neglect*, institutional medicine may be said to neglect patients in two fundamental ways. First, it over-emphasizes the biomedical model to the point that it often neglects and or ignores the human side of illness and suffering. Although this insight has been a major concern of medical humanities scholarship for the past thirty years, the biomedical model continues to reign supreme in medicine with very little in the way of effective counterbalance.[2] Second, institutional medicine neglects patients by failing to care for and meaningfully research social variables, which have been and remain the most important determinants to health. Throughout much of the world, poverty and social injustice are the leading causes of health problems (World Health Organization, 1995; Farmer, 2005). And even among over-industrialized, over-consumptive, and over-corporatized nations, the leading cause of health problems are social: stress, early life traumas, unsafe workplaces, unemployment, lack of social support, addiction, poor food quality, dangerous transportation systems and growing social gradients (World Health Organization, 1998). Medicine fails to adequately research and intervene in all of these issues, and as a consequence, effectively neglects millions of patients caught up in the suffering, morbidity, and mortality caused by these social issues.

The *abuse* side of institutional medicine comes from the way patients are harmed. While largely silent on issues social injustice and human suffering, contemporary medicine *is* highly outspoken in its advocacy of specialized biotechnological interventions. These high tech, high cost, and usually high corporate interventions may sometimes be helpful, but all too often they are hurtful. They divert monetary resources that could be applied to other solutions, and they place patients at serious risk of bodily damage (Callahan, 1998; Starfield, 2000). Current estimates make a compelling case that medical interventions are a leading cause of death in the U.S. Public health scholar Barbara Starfield estimates that the combined effect of medical errors and adverse effects in the United States are as follows:

- 12,000 deaths/year from unnecessary surgery
- 7000 deaths/year from medication errors in hospitals
- 20,000 deaths/year from other errors in hospitals
- 80,000 deaths/year from nosocomial infections in hospitals
- 106,000 deaths/year from nonerror, adverse effects of medications.

That comes to a total to 225,000 deaths per year from iatrogenic causes, which constitutes the third leading cause of death in the United States just after heart disease and cancer (Starfield, 2000, p. 484).

And if that were not bad enough, the last thing one sees focusing upstream may be the most unfaceable insight of them all: medicine's neglect and abuse of patients is not an accident, but a direct outcome of the way medicine has been set up. But how can this be? Medicine, by all manifest accounts, is a beneficent institution. The answer comes back to the discourses (language, rules, norms, practices, and institutions) of medicine. These discourses do not appear magically or come from nowhere. Unlike the weather, they are not forced by the hand of nature. Instead, the dominant discourses of medicine come from the leadership of medicine and the corporations that sustain it. This leadership may be unconscious of the social effects of their individual decisions, and they may work through consumer consensus rather than direct force, but there is no escaping that the discourse of medicine comes primarily from these leaders (Morgan, 1998). It comes from the CEOs of hospitals, pharmaceuticals, biotech companies, and the health insurance industry. It comes from department chairs of major academic health centers, from the directors of the National Institutes of Health, from the editors and contributors of the leading journals, and from the leaders of major medical organizations and lobbying groups. In short, a sociological imagination reveals that medical discursive priorities are constructed, sustained, and developed by the leaders of contemporary institutions.

This concern and realization over where the discourses of institutional medicine come from is precisely where the second incommensurability shows up in the *AJOB* issue. Wear and Kuczewski call for more democratic knowledge making in medicine, and they focus their concern on the participatory role medical students and residents could have in creating the discourse of medical professionalism. But Wear and Kuczewski's idea that students and residents participate in knowledge making (rather than simply knowledge learning) went over very poorly with most respondents. Indeed, many respondents were simply aghast at the idea. Students and residents, they decried, cannot tell us about professionalism. Professionalism curricula can only come from the experts. For most of the respondents, the idea that quality knowledge comes from qualified experts is unassailable. But here again there is a tremendous incommensurability. From within the logic of a sociological imagination, the perspective shifts completely. That is, within the sociological imagination, the notion that expert knowledge making must be accountable to democracy has become so obvious to be a kind of common place (Harding, 1991; Sclove, 1995; Kleinman, 2000; Guston, 2002).

From this perspective it seems clear that without a more democratic knowledge making process, the discourse of institutional medicine will not respond to its current problems. It will not, in other words, meaningfully respond to its neglect and abuse of patients. Despite all of their expertise, medical leaders are unlikely to spot the problems within contemporary medical institutions; that is, they benefit too much from the current priorities of medicine to change. As Marcia Angell points out with regard to the relationship between medicine and the pharmaceutical industry (just one of the many powerful interests within medicine today):

> Over the past two decades the pharmaceutical industry has moved very far from its original high purpose of discovering and producing useful new drugs. Now primarily a marketing machine to sell drugs of dubious benefit, the industry uses its wealth and power to co-opt every institution that might stand in its way, including the U.S. Congress, the FDA, academic medical centers, and the medical profession itself. (Angell, 2004)

Angell's insight makes it clear that the leaders of medicine will not change by themselves. They will only change if they are held more democratically responsive to different constituents. They will change only if they become less accountable to commercial profit motives and more accountable to their main constituents—their patients and their trainees.

INSTITUTIONAL MEDICINE IS MEDICAL PROFESSIONALISM'S WORST ENEMY

The great irony of this discursive analysis is that if you bring these two incommensurabilities together, and if you seriously focus upstream on institutional medicine, you realize how unlikely it is that contemporary medicine will ever, or at least any time soon, be very professional. Indeed, just the opposite is true: institutional medicine is paradoxically a major impediment to the individual physician achieving the goals of professionalism. This situation is likely to get worse before it gets better. Medical knowledge making shows no signs of opening up to democratic practices. When and if the profession of medicine does change, it will be the result of major activism. In the mean time, students must continue to study medicine and teachers must continue to teach it.

So, what is to be done? How can teachers and students respond to this paradoxical situation? One could argue, as Wear and Kuczewski effectively do, that teaching professionalism is part of the problem rather than part of the solution. For Wear and Kuczewski, the professionalism movement covers over and effaces the conflicts inherent in institutional medicine. The professionalism movement is filled with empty abstractions and pays too little attention to social issues. The professionalism movement, in effect, blames the victims—individual students and practitioners—for the system of medicine's inability and unwillingness to deal with structural problems and conflicts. The result is a discourse on professionalism that works as a ruse. Leaders of medical systems and medical organizations can point to the grand ideals of professionalism while doing very little to change the medical system's own barriers to living up to those ideals.

But I would argue that the professionalism movement is salvageable if we rework the discourse of professionalism to include a meaningful distinction between individual physicians and the institutions of medicine. From my discursive analysis, the crux of the conflict is this: the values of the professionalism movement and those of the medicine as an institution are too often in conflict. A way out of this conflict would be to make a sharp distinction between the institution of medicine as a *social* phenomenon and the professionalism movement as largely focused on *individual* physicians. At present, this distinction between the institutions of medicine and individual doctors is not reliably being made, resulting in a fundamental discursive silence in the language of professionalism.

This discursive silence exists on both sides of the conflicts and incommensurability addressed above. It creates a discourse of professionalism that foregrounds the qualities of responsibility, virtue, caring, and ethics—the essential qualities of professionalism—for individual physicians, but leaves mute these very same qualities for the institutions of medicine as a whole. Remarkably, the discourse of professionalism has no meaningful language for talking about "the profession" understood as the larger institutions of medicine within which individual physicians practice.

To see how this works consider the way today's discourse of professionalism focuses on and even demands that individual physicians live up to a series of standards. Although the standards come in different forms, they are usually variations of those put out by the Accreditation Council on

Graduate Medical Education (ACGME) and the American Board of Medical Specialties (ABMS). Their 2000 *ACGME/ABMS Outcome Project* states that residents are expected to "demonstrate respect, compassion, and integrity: a responsiveness to the needs of patients and society that supersedes self-interest: accountability to patients, society, and the profession, and a commitment to excellence and on-going professional development" (cited in Wear & Kuczewski, 2004, p. 2).

Paradoxically, although these standards have wide consensus among medical educators, a major block to achieving these standards is the profession of medicine itself. When ACGME/ABMS says that physicians should be "responsive to the needs of patients, society, and the profession," they give physicians a proverbial double bind because the interests of patients, society, and the profession of medicine are often in conflict. When individual physicians are responsive to the needs of patients and society, they too often find themselves being unresponsive the interests of profession. Institutional medicine's neglect and abuse of patients discussed earlier means that to be responsive to patients and society, individual physicians must often struggle against the dominant trends within the profession.

This is clearly a conundrum, but it is not irremediable. If we bring to the discourse of professionalism a meaningful distinction between the *individual* physician and the *social institution* of medicine, the individual physician's "responsiveness" to the profession could well include a struggle against deeply problematic trends within the profession. In this light, part of the task of individual physicians would be to help the institution of medicine bring out its most worthy characteristics: to help it curb its appetite for an ever increased slice of the GNP, to help it work within limits and toward sustainability, to help it shift some of its research efforts and social weight from profits to resolution of social causes of human suffering, and to help it generate more democratic knowledge making practices. These are all invaluable forms of responsiveness to the profession.[3] But, to make this move, young physicians need a clear distinction between themselves and the larger institution of medicine, and they need a deep understanding of contemporary critiques of the profession they are entering. They need to know they are joining a profession that is sometimes a route to health, but is all too often a nemesis to health.[4]

TEACHING THE CONFLICTS

In short, individual students and practitioners of medicine need to be taught the conflicts surrounding the institutions of medicine. I borrow the phrase "teach the conflicts" from Gerald Graff, a professor of English and education whose key work in this domain is titled *Beyond the Culture Wars: How Teaching the Conflicts Can Revitalize American Education*. Graff argues that teachers benefit from adopting a conflict model for their pedagogic practices, a model that recognizes, accepts, and teaches the tensions within higher education (Graff, 1992). These insights are born out of the climate of tremendous conflicts surrounding the traditional canon of "great works" and the role of theory in humanities education. Graff concludes that for teachers and students, these cultural wars that often pit so-called "traditional values" against so-called "multicultural values" should not be seen as a sign of crisis as much as moment of opportunity.

Graff explains how pedagogic practice in the humanities can make fertile use of this debate, and how the "culture wars" can be a means to make education better, as crucial questions are raised, analyzed, and debated. Of course, bringing these crucial questions to the classroom will not resolve them in a way satisfactory to the warring parties. The only solution that would fully satisfy staunch defenders of one position or another would be that all other positions be relegated to the margins as unimportant, misguided, or worse, delusional ideology. But, as Graff puts it, no matter what our positions we must accept that unconditional surrender, or full curricular control, is not a winnable prize. Rather than trying to win the not winnable, and rather than teaching as if all other positions were misguided, educators should stage the debates and involve students in them. Educators should expose students to historical and contemporary struggles in medicine and help them to understand and articulate why these issues matter so they can gauge where they stand themselves. By teaching the conflicts, Graff argues that education takes a more democratic turn, based on free exchange of ideas and recognition that the alternative is an impasse.

Francis Oakly, in his book *Community of Learning: The American College and the Liberal Arts Tradition* (1992), praises Graff for prompting faculty and students to address "stubbornly intractable disagreements directly" (p. 159). Oakly recognizes the risk that this pedagogic practice may confuse students, but points out that students are already confused as they move from one isolated course or discipline to another, maneuvering "among radically divergent theories of knowledge without being fully conscious of so doing, and without getting adequate help in the process" (p. 161). Using Graff's work as a guide, Oakly argues that foregrounding the conflicts deepens and furthers the education of students, because it demonstrates for both faculty and students the necessity of facing conflicts directly. And it models an intellectual exploration where all perspectives are given serious attention in the context of a generous and civil discussion.

Graff's "teaching the conflicts" approach provides tremendous assistance to the medical professionalism debate. The advent of medical professionalism movement, like the "culture wars" in the humanities, comes in a time of tremendous tension and conflict surrounding the institution of medicine. Critics of professionalism such as Wear and Kuczewski argue that the movement covers over these conflicts. Advocates of professionalism believe the movement improves these conflicts by providing individual physicians with abstract ideals to guide their action and behavior. The way out of this discursive impasse is to make a clear distinction between individual practitioners and medical institutions. Once that distinction is clear, professionalism educators can engage the individual students in the conflicts regarding today's medical institutions, which encourages them to develop a sense of where they stand with regard to current institutions, to develop their own positions, and to decide where they will put a shoulder to the wheel of defining and creating tomorrow's health care system.

In conclusion, I argue that the medical professionalism movement can continue to inspire physicians in training to live up to the goals and standards of professionalism. But this will only be meaningful if the professionalism movement also helps students understand the ways institutional medicine can be a powerful hindrance to the goals of professionalism. For the professionalism movement to work, students need to understand the conflicts embedded in the profession they are entering, and they need exposure to critical scholarship that looks upstream to expose the deep problems with contemporary medical systems. Students need to recognize the fundamental contradictions between institutional medicine and the individual values of professionalism. They need to see that a profession that emphasizes expert driven, high tech, high cost interventions at the expense of humane primary care, social justice, and democratic inquiry cannot be seen as altruistic, knowledgeable, ethical, or dutiful. Once they understand these contradictions, students can better navigate the double binds involved, and they can better participate in crafting the humane and democratic medical institutions of tomorrow.

ENDNOTES

[1]   I use the phrase "institutional medicine" to include medical research, education, and delivery systems, along with the insurance, pharmaceutical, and biotech corporations that influence and sustain them.

[2]   See Margaret Edson's Pulitzer prize winning play *Wit* for a dramatization of institutional medicine's neglect of the human dimensions of illness (Edson, 1993). Also see Eric Cassell's book *Doctoring: The Nature of Primary Care Medicine* for an extended discussion of the difficulties medicine has in taking seriously the subjective dimensions of the patient as person (Cassell, 1997).

[3]   For some examples of public medical intellectuals and medical scholars who have taken on this kind of task see: "Medical Intellectuals: Resisting Medical Orientalism" (Aull and Lewis, 2004). See also the health care group "No Free Lunch" started by New York City internist Bob Goodman, M.D. (www.nofreelunch.org). No Free Lunch works to counter excessive promotional hype coming from pharmaceuticals, which can severely interfere with best medical practices. In addition, see the British "Critical Psychiatry Network" (www.critpsynet.freeuk.com). This network of psychiatrists work to intervene and to join with activist efforts against some of the worst features of contemporary British psychiatry. As CPN puts it in their position statement:
We believe that there is a need to resist attempts to make psychiatry *more* coercive. In its attempts to take forward this agenda, the Network has:
--Made clear its opposition to compulsory treatment in evidence submitted to the Government's Scoping Group set up to review the Mental Health Act.
--Submitted evidence to the Government, arguing against the idea of preventive detention.
--Carried out a survey of senior English psychiatrists to seek their views about preventive detention.
--Worked closely with other groups, coordinated by MIND, in trying to influence government policy. (http://www.critpsynet.freeuk.com/position.htm).

[4]   In this vein, the connection between the professionalism movement and the "white coat ceremony" seems particularly problematic. The white coat ceremony is a recently devised ritual within medical schools where students are ceremoniously draped in "the white coat" to symbolize the purity and goodness of the profession they are about to enter (Wear, 1998). From the perspective of the deep problems with today's institution of medicine, it would perhaps make more sense for the students to engage in a "tattered coat ceremony." Part of the ritual might involve the students taking the coat off and spending time mending the tears. The tattered coat could symbolize the deep problems within the institution of medicine and the mending exercise could symbolize the student's role in improving the profession.

REFERENCES

Angell, M. (2004). The truth about drug companies. Retrieved August 29, 2004 from http://www.nybooks.com/articles/17244
Aull, F. & Lewis, B. (2004). Medical intellectuals: Resisting medical orientalism. *Journal of medical humanities, 25*(2): 87-108.

Bauman, Z. (1990). *Modernity and ambivalence.* Cambridge, England: Polity Press.

Callahan, D. (1998). *False hopes: Why America's quest for perfect health is a recipe for failure.* New York: Simon and Shuster.

Cassell, E. (1997). *Doctoring: The nature of primary care.* Oxford: Oxford University Press.

Edson, M. (1993). *Wit.* New York: Faber and Faber, Inc.

Farmer, P. (2005). *Pathologies of power: Health, human rights, and the new war on the poor.* Berkeley: University of California Press.

Graff, G. (1992). *Beyond the culture wars: How teaching the conflicts can revitalize American education.* New York: Norton.

Groth, H. (1982) Interpretation for Freud and Heidegger. *International Review of Psychoanalysis. 9,* 67-74.

Guston, D. (2002). The regulatory environment for science: Does democracy trump science? In A. Teich et al. (Eds.), *AAAS science and policy yearbook.* New York: American Association for the Advancement of Science.

Harding, S. (1991). *Whose science? Whose knowledge? Thinking from women's lives.* Ithaca, NY: Cornell University Press.

Kleinman, D.L. (Ed.). (2000). *Science, technology, and democracy.* Albany: State University of New York Press.

Lewis, B. (in press). *Moving beyond Prozac, DSM, and the new psychiatry: Birth of postpsychiatry.* Ann Arbor: University of Michigan Press.

Mills, C.W. (1959). *The sociological imagination.* London: Oxford University Press.

McKinlay, J. (2001). A case for refocusing upstream: The political economy of illness. In P. Conrad (Ed.), *The sociology of health and illness* (pp. 516-529). New York: Worth.

Morgan, K. P. (1998). Contested bodies, contested knowledges: Women, health, and the politics of medicalization. In S. Sherwin (Ed.), *The politics of women's health: Exploring agency and autonomy* (pp. 83-122). Philadelphia: Temple University Press.

Oakly, F. (1992) *Community of learning: The American college and the liberal arts tradition.* New York. Oxford University Press.

Sclove, R. (1995). *Democracy and technology.* New York: The Guilford Press.

Shirley, J., & Padgett, S. (2004). Professionalism and discourse: But wait, there's more! *American Journal of Bioethics. 4*(2): 36-38.

Starfield, B. (2000). Is U.S. health really the best in the world? *Journal of the American Medical Association.* 284 (4), 483-5.

Wear, D. (1998). On white coats and professional development: The formal and the hidden curriculum. *Annals of Internal Medicine, 129,* 734-737.

Wear, D. & Kuczewski, M. (2004). The professionalism movement: Can we pause? *American Journal of Bioethics, 4*(2), 1-10.

World Health Organization. (1995). *Bridging the gaps.* Geneva: World Health Organization.

World Health Organization. (1998). *Social determinants of health: The solid facts.* Geneva: World Health Organization.

Part Three

ASSESSING PROFESSIONALISM

Chapter 9

EDUCATING FOR PROFESSIONALISM AT INDIANA UNIVERSITY SCHOOL OF MEDICINE
Feet on the Ground and Fresh Eyes

Thomas S. Inui with Ann H. Cottingham, Richard M. Frankel, Debra K. Litzelman, David L. Mossbarger, Anthony L. Suchman, T. Robert Vu, Penelope R. Williamson
Indiana University School of Medicine and Regenstrief Institute, Inc.

> *"I watched a member of the housestaff give a rather cursory consent for a central line placement. Although the patient medically needed the line, the procedure was barely explained to the patient, and the patient may not have even been competent. In addition the nursing staff was pushing the house staff to put in the central line."* A third-year medical student, Indiana University School of Medicine, 2004.

In this chapter, we explore the meaning of professionalism in an historical and social context and discuss means by which medical schools as complex organizations might reinvigorate education for professionalism. We next describe efforts at Indiana University School of Medicine (IUSM) to integrate (1) a highly specified formal curriculum with (2) student learning about professional values from their own experience (the informal curriculum). Turning to the question of how organizational change processes might effectively shape the environment in which students become physicians, we discuss Stacey's (2000) new theory—Complex Responsive Processes of Relating—that undergirds our attempts to change the culture of a large medical school and, therefore, align the formal and the informal curricula at IUSM. We conclude with some thoughts about the intersection of personal, professional and organizational development.

In an historical context, "professionalism" has had various meanings at different times in North America (Sullivan, 1995). About a century ago, "professional" literally denoted someone who was *paid* for what s/he did. Bobby Jones, for example, was not a "professional golfer," though he was the very best golfer of his era. In spite of his excellence, he remained an amateur and was, therefore, never considered to be a professional. At other times in our history, especially as the sociologist Parsons (1968) explored the concept, professional came to mean *learned* and *self-regulating*. Professionals could restrict entry into a field of work, essentially creating a monopoly, because no other element of the general society could judge the performance or quality of individuals within such a technically complex field. In recent times, the word "professional" in general usage typically refers to individuals who claim to be truly excellent at what they do, whether or not there is any external standard against which to judge the quality of their work or work product. Perusing the yellow pages of any telephone directory, for example, uncovers *professional* painters, *professional* homebuilders, *professional* movers, and others.

Schools of medicine in our day are focused, as perhaps medicine at large is, on reclaiming the status of a learned profession for physicians as a work group within our society (Inui, 2003). This reclamation may be especially important today because of the many sources of distress in our field stemming from high expense, visible errors, a general impression that physicians are both expensive and personally wealthy, and the "cold fusion" of clinical medicine with commercial enterprise as for-profit insurance plans and institutions emerge, often lead by physician executives. Medicine and commercialism have become co-mingled.

In the midst of this co-mingling of social sectors, it may be important for medicine to re-establish itself as a trustworthy work group within our society. Though individual personal physicians are generally rated as trustworthy by their patients, public trust has dramatically declined for physicians at large (Hall, Dugan, Zheng, & Mishra, 2001). Much of what physicians can accomplish hinges on having this trust, and trustworthy professions are especially needed by our general society. Few other institutions are implicitly trusted and admired by our citizenry, as Eliot Freidson (2001) has pointed out. American society is disinclined to trust political institutions, given disturbing experiences with the presidency and taints of corruption in our national legislature. Trust of organized religion has been eroded by revelations of priests' sexual abuse of members of the Catholic Church, including children. Multinational corporations, certainly a major economic force on the American scene, are not to be trusted in the era of corruption at Enron, Global Crossing, and other instances of corporate self-dealing to the disadvantage of stockholders and the public.

While reestablishing professionalism in medicine may be critically important, there is no clear-cut understanding of how this might be done. Major professional associations like the American College of Physicians and American Society of Internal Medicine (ACP-ASIM), the European Federation of Internal Medicine, and certifying bodies such as the American Board of Internal Medicine, acting within their established spheres of influence and operations, have together emphasized the importance of continuing professional development and recertification. Members of the Medical Professionalism Project deliberated, adopted, and promulgated a Professional Charter, a statement of principles, values, and implied social accountability (Members of the Medical Professionalism Project, 2002). The National Board of Medical Examiners (2004) has reintroduced a Clinical Skills Examination as a required component of the basic licensing examination that emphasizes responsive communication with patients as a basic clinical competency and a critical domain of performance separate from knowledge of biomedical sciences (National Board of Medical Examiners, 2002). The profession is perhaps especially concerned about establishing a construct of professionalism and professional values for students of medicine, who at present seem to be cynical about the field and the behaviors of practitioners of medicine, even about the physicians within the academic medical center environment, i.e. the faculty. The origin of this cynicism may not be a mystery (Testerman, Morton, Loo, Worthley, & Lamberton, 1996). Medical center faculty members teach an ideal set of values and behaviors in the classroom, but the students see many of these ideals abridged or violated in academic medical center-based practice. Therefore, they understand from their own experience that medicine may literally be a field in which "we say one thing and then do another."

How can this unfortunate situation be rectified? In his monograph *A Flag in the Wind: Educating for Professionalism in Medicine*, Inui (2003) outlines a variety of ways of proceeding to create organizational change in order to align the "hidden" or informal curriculum (the slice of academic medical center life that students experience) with the formal curriculum (what we teach in the classroom). Some of his "action agenda" options are cited in Table 1.

Table I. Enhancing Education for Professionalism: Selected Action Agenda Examples

---

Enhance the recognition of the relevance of professionalism to key institutional roles and accountabilities.

- Make explicit the connection between professional values/behaviors and leadership development for Deans, Chairs, Chief residents
- Deans' actions to put professionalism, exemplary behaviors, monitoring, improvement, and feedback on the organizational agenda for performance evaluation and compensation

Make explicit the role of professionalism in organizational performance and management.

- Forge and implement a meaningful organizational 'code of ethics'
- Integrate professional norms for behavior into institutional missions, operations (e.g. with patient and staff reporting, feedback, hotlines)

Make explicit the role of professionalism in trainee/physician/program performance within the organization.

- Make explicit a focus on a candidate's history of meaningful service to others a component of medical school and residency applications (e.g. essay, interview)
- Measure and report meaningful content in the broad domain of professional qualities for the dean's assessment letter
- Discuss the medical school code of conduct (with focus groups of patients, staff, and faculty) annually in a process that focuses on a few specific, current challenges

Enhance resources for continued learning and professional development in the hidden curriculum.

- Model positive professional behavior in the teacher/learner relationship
- Conduct morbidity and mortality conferences that avoid shame and humiliation, teach how to frame 'medical errors' constructively, and lead on to continuous improvement

Promote resources that make explicit the link between personal and professional growth and development.

- Qualitative methods (e.g. semi-structured debriefings) to assess "what's being learned?" in contradistinction to "what's being taught"
- Patient and peer ratings of physician performance used for continuing professional development, especially those focused on physician trustworthiness and interpersonal skills
- Small group teaching/learning that includes, as a standard feature of group process, feedback on behaviors within the group that facilitate or inhibit individual and group functioning

While all these alternative actions may each be reasonable options for influencing the environment in which our students become physicians, the sheer number of specific strategies can be daunting to contemplate. Within a large organization, only a few might seem feasible. Compounding this difficulty is the observation that responsibility for special initiatives such as these is often assigned to a school committee (e.g. the admissions or curriculum committee), where a few persons are asked to contemplate assuming new responsibilities outside of their "day jobs" but have limited time and minimal staff support. The organizational objective is nevertheless compelling. If cynicism is to be avoided and strong, integrated and consistent learning is to occur, we need to *align* the formal and informal curricula.

Suppose, under these circumstances and with this aim in mind, the good-willed committee chooses to start with just one action step. Could any specific action have a significant, systemic effect on the larger organization? From an organizational development "theory of action" perspective, how might such a larger effect materialize? Since many individuals in academic medical centers do not have a strong educational orientation or sense of mission, but instead focus narrowly on research or clinical practice activities, how could the actions of a few faculty members affect the larger organizational environment and many others?

At Indiana University School of Medicine, we have taken these challenges in hand and are explicitly attempting to align the formal and informal curricula to enhance student and faculty professional development. What follows is an explication of our approach and theory of action.

PROFESSIONALISM—AN IUSM CORE COMPETENCY OBJECTIVE

At IUSM, education for professionalism takes place in the context of a competency-directed general curriculum, within which professionalism is identified as one of nine core competencies to be acquired in the course of each student's four-year experience (Indiana University School of Medicine, 1996). Growth and development in professionalism, like in the other competencies, is considered to be an explicit objective of every required experience a student has at IUSM.

The IUSM statewide Professionalism Competency Director, Richard Frankel, identifies six core elements of professionalism:

- Altruism
- Responsibility and accountability
- Leadership
- Caring, compassion
- Honor and integrity
- Self-correction

The overall aim of the professionalism competency is to inculcate within the IUSM graduate the values, understanding, skills and behaviors of professionalism that will serve them and the public well in their day-to-day roles as physicians.   For example, accountability for self-correction is foundational to the practice of medicine (Cruess, Johnston, & Cruess, 2004). The IUSM curriculum is consciously constructed to foster this ability in our students.   We have developed a series of learning experiences that require students to observe, reflect, and comment on the behaviors, interchanges and activities that they see and participate in every day.   As students practice the process of self-correction over the four year period of their undergraduate education, our goal is that this process will stimulate their own professional development and will provide them a heightened awareness and heightened level of comfort with self-correction as an essential part of their professional obligations.

The operational definition of competency in professionalism is articulated as a set of specific behavioral objectives (Indiana University School of Medicine, 1996).   It is our aim to produce physicians who will:

A. Behave professionally
- Be responsible, reliable, and dependable
- Demonstrate personal integrity, honesty, and self-discipline
- Project a professional image in manner, dress, grooming, and interpersonal relationships that is consistent with the medical profession's accepted contemporary standards in the community
- Recognize personal limitations and biases, whether they are intellectual, physical, or emotional, and seek additional help/consultation where appropriate
- Demonstrate the professional and emotional maturity to take appropriate steps to resolve tensions and conflicts which occur among professional, personal, and family responsibilities, seeking professional help if necessary
- Demonstrate the ability to exercise sound judgment and function under pressure

B. Interact effectively with the patient

- Treat the patient as a person, not a disease, realizing that the person who is ill is more important as an individual and as a member of his/her social group than is the illness that person has.
- Be aware of and accept that the patient is a person with important values, goals, and concerns, who lives in a particular family/community context, and that these factors have a significant impact on the disease process, the treatment of disease, and the patient's ability to cooperate in the management of these problems
- Respect the patient's rights and privacy
- Adopt a professional manner in each patient encounter in a way that allows each patient to feel he/she has received satisfactory, empathetic professional service
- Recognize the following issues that could affect the patient's management and modify management as appropriate:
  a) Legal issues
  b) Ethical issues (each as informed consent, truth telling, malpractice)
  c) Conflict of values between the patient and the community
  d) Psychosocial issues
  e) Religious issues

C. Interact effectively with the entire health-care team, other health professionals, and community professionals
- Utilize the expertise of other professionals and experts, as appropriate, in the care of the patient, being aware of their particular abilities, skills, and role in health-care delivery
- Know how to obtain this additional help
- Be willing to both receive and give information and advice from and to other health-care professionals in everyday work with patients and in health-care settings
- Work cooperatively with other professionals as members of a team in patient care
- Use appropriate steps in dealing with unethical behavior by other members of the health-care team

D. Demonstrate leadership and motivation
E. Coordinate the management of the patient's problem
F. Mentor junior members of the health care team

Every course at IUSM has a professionalism objective. In a basic science course, the professional value, knowledge, and behaviors may be expressed in actions that are part of small-group exercises where good preparation, support of collaborative learning, and asking for or getting help may express leadership, integrity, altruism, self-correction and other professional behaviors. In the clinical clerkships that come later in the curriculum, actions with other members of the clinical team or with patients and their families, express the same values in a different context.

The evaluation of student growth and development in professionalism, as well as feedback to students on their progress in this competency, is similarly suffused throughout the four-year curriculum. Currently we evaluate progress in professionalism:

• In the first year, by small group facilitators and preceptors in Introduction to Clinical Medicine (ICM) I and Concepts of Health and Disease.
• In the second year, by small group preceptors in ICM II and General Pathology.
• In the Systemic Pathology course in second year, an assessment of a written report and oral presentation of three autopsy cases.
• In the third year Medicine Clerkship, using unannounced standardized patients who fill out a checklist that includes professionalism behaviors, and on the basis of professionalism logs that students fill out electronically and share with one another in a facilitated small group discussion.
• In the third year Medicine/Neurology/Psychiatry intersession, through progressive student narratives, small group discussion, and role plays.
• In the Family Medicine Clerkship, using a checklist of professional behaviors.
• In the Pediatric Clerkship, using a checklist of behaviors and parents' comments about the students' professionalism in caring for their hospitalized children.

In addition to specifying core elements and assessment methods, IUSM attempts to weave student experiences in the informal curriculum into the formal curriculum (Figure 1) for the purposes of individual and community reflection, dialogue, and professional growth. IUSM community members' narratives are generated by student, staff, and faculty journals, parents of pediatric patients, and notes from interviews conducted among IUSM community members that promote dialogue about what is working well within the organization's Relationship-Centered Care Initiative (Suchman, et. al, 2004). These narratives are mined for competency-relevant content that can be used as core content for student educational materials and faculty development programs. An educational quality improvement strategy, centered in IUSM's Office of Medical Education and Curricular Affairs, assures use of these materials in the curriculum as well as community activities of conscious reflection and dialogue that in turn shape the hidden curriculum (Suchman et. al, 2004; Inui, 2004).

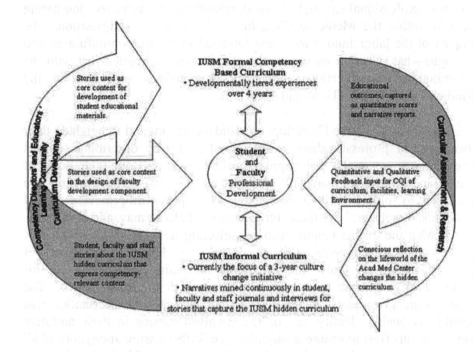

Figure I. Aligning the IUSM Formal and Informal Competency Based Curriculum

AN EXAMPLE OF MINING THE INFORMAL CURRICULUM

In 2003, Indiana University School of Medicine was one of ten North American medical schools selected by the American Medical Association (AMA) to design innovative methods for teaching and assessing the competency behaviors that constitute professionalism. This partnership between the 10 selected medical schools and the AMA is known as the STEP (Strategies for Teaching and Evaluating Professionalism) Program. The grant has catalyzed a significant advance in our institution's undergraduate competency curriculum in professionalism. Wanting to align experiential learning with classroom teaching, we focused our efforts on two innovative teaching interventions during the students' rotation through the Medicine Clerkship: (1) the use of unannounced standardized patients in ambulatory clinic settings to evaluate and teach medical students selected issues of professionalism, and (2) the development of a reflective journaling activity within the Medicine Clerkship. Of these two interventions, the impact of the latter innovation—one intended to enhance mindfulness and dialogue—has clearly surpassed the former and delighted us with its contributions to educational enhancement activities well beyond the Medicine Clerkship at IUSM and elsewhere.

During the Medicine Clerkship, our students are invited to heighten their awareness of professionalism as embodied action by describing seminal events (large or small) that express professionalism (from their point of view) and have been part of their own experiences. These events are recorded as online written narratives in a password-protected IUSM educational website. To these little stories, students may add reflections about what the events taught them by selecting items from a checklist of professionalism elements (drawn from the NBME definition of professionalism). Only the Medicine Clerkship Director and his administrative assistant have complete access to these online entries. The students are given strict instructions to not include any information that would personally identify any of the involved parties in their narrative entries, in an effort to ensure anonymity. To further ensure anonymity of all involved parties, including the students themselves, the Medicine Clerkship Director reviews every student narrative entry to make any necessary edits and/or deletions of those entries that may compromise anonymity. Each month, the edited and anonymous journal narratives are printed and distributed to the students for small group reflection and discussion sessions with an expert faculty facilitator. In these sessions, students are invited to choose stories they would like to read aloud to their peers. A student reader is asked why s/he chose the narrative, and then the discussion is opened to a dialogue among all present. The discussions are far-reaching: "Is this a common event? Can you explain why this happens? What is it about the people in this story that makes this happen? What is it about the circumstance or setting that makes this possible? How could this kind of event happen less often? More often?" After the session, the hard copies are all collected and destroyed to further ensure student anonymity.

The STEP narratives often contain such powerful representations of professionalism and descriptions of role models in action (good or bad) that they have become part of the formal curriculum of the Medicine Clerkship. A similar journaling process will be adopted by the Surgery Clerkship in June 2005. From our review of the student narratives thus far, we can report that students are astute observers of both professional and unprofessional behaviors that occur around them. Because they are not yet inured to many of the potentially upsetting interactions that occur among people (doctors, nurses, patients, family members, staff) in clinical settings, they have a sensibility that lies somewhere between fully formed clinicians and lay persons. The content of their narratives varies from dispassionate observation, to reporting with explicit emotional content (e.g., admiration, disappointment, inspiration), to observation with varying degrees of self-reflection and learning.

Here is an example of a relatively dispassionate observation:

"I was following a cardiologist who would not abandon his terminal patients even if medically he could no longer do anything for them. He would take a house call and be with the patient until the last day of their lives. He would state 'It is criminal to abandon your patient—even if there is no cure, there still may be healing.'" On the list of professional elements, this student checked: Altruism; Responsibility and Accountability; Excellence and Scholarship; Respect; Caring, Compassion, and Communication.

Many narratives express much more overt student affect:

"A resident was performing a thoracentesis on a patient who had had a prolonged hospital stay with multiple complications. The patient was resistant to the procedure because he was tired of being 'stuck so much.' The resident, who did not appear particularly confident himself, instructed the intern on how to perform the procedure in front of the patient. The patient, who already made it clear he did not want someone inexperienced to be 'poking me,' was even more apprehensive after the tutorial. After multiple attempts, the intern failed to obtain pleural fluid. The resident then attempted and was successful. The resident then chided the patient for not being cooperative by saying 'And you didn't think we'd get it, did you? Well, look here.' And he showed the patient the vacutainer bottle. I felt the patient was made to feel like a guinea pig and then was belittled for complaining about the pain. Neither of the residents were empathetic to the patient and treated him like a bag of flour." This student checked: Caring, Compassion, and Communication.

"Our team and the ICU team were rounding and we all entered a patient's room. There were at least 15 of us in the room. Our teams spoke about the patient, examined him, adjusted the ventilator setting, and then left— all oblivious to the family member who was in the room the entire time. After we had all left, I noticed that the intern—who had just started the service that morning—kneeled down beside the patient's wife and began explaining what the team had just done. No one else noticed what she had done, but I was very impressed by her behavior." This student checked: Caring, Compassion, and Communication.

Still other narratives contain explicit self-reflection and/or comments on learning:

"A fourth-year student and I contacted the family of a dying patient and, rather than waiting for them to arrive, we entered the patient's room to inform her that her sister said 'she loves you.' The patient, catching her breath, replied 'I love her, too.' And at that point, I realized that our words were likely much more beneficial than any of the dozens of medicines on board as the patient instantly became calm and seemed at peace." This student checked: Respect; Honor and Integrity; Caring, Compassion, and Communication.

"An obese patient had to have his groin examined. There was a very strong odor to which the doctor almost got sick. He told the patient how bad it smelled. I would have done my best to make it through the exam but not make the patient feel any worse about the smell because he knew about the smell but could not do anything about it." This student checked: Respect; Caring, Compassion, and Communication.

"One of the patients I'm taking care of is a solely French-speaking man from West Africa. Fortunately, his sister stays in the room with him and helps to translate. But my resident still has never yet directly communicated or made much in the way of eye contact with the patient. All questions go the sister; sometimes it's like the patient's not even there.

When I've gone to see the patient alone I find myself falling into this trap. It's quite awkward when you can't directly communicate, so I've at least tried non-verbal communication—e.g., eye contact, therapeutic touch, etc., and truthfully I think the patient is responding better to that."

This student checked: Respect; Caring, Compassion, and Communication.

The STEP narratives communicate such rich content of relevance to professionalism, that it is often difficult to complete a discussion of more than two stories in a one-hour small group session. It is our hope and expectation that these stories and discussions will create mindfulness of professionalism among our students, and also among our faculty and housestaff. We have begun to use these journal narratives in anonymous, aggregate, and edited format, once the students have graduated from medical school, to provide feedback to our faculty and residents in various venues (such as faculty development workshops and departmental grand rounds) in an effort to improve teaching and role modeling of professionalism through better self-awareness of all in the informal curriculum. On the basis of discussions we have had with students thus far, we believe that we have created a safe environment for observations and reflections about professionalism at IUSM to be shared freely, if anonymously, thereby fostering organizational change through use of their "fresh eyes" and reflective capacity.

It has also been exciting, as the process of gathering and discussing STEP narratives in the Medicine Clerkship has matured, to see the other activities at IUSM that this project and its narratives have stimulated and supported.

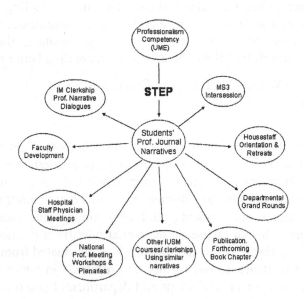

Figure 1. Impact of STEP Student Narratives at Indiana University School of Medicine

   To our delight, the STEP narratives have begun to be used widely (Figure 2, starting at "1 o'clock" and continuing clockwise) as:

- discussion triggers for a new third-year intersession on professionalism
- reminders to new interns of how they serve as role models
- examples in departmental grand rounds discussions of professionalism and ACGME requirements for an explicit professionalism curriculum in residency
- writing for publication
- models for other clerkships adopting this process at IUSM
- seminal events for various organizations' workshops on professionalism and humanism
- examples for hospital staff deliberations on patient expectations, professional standards, and malpractice risk
- content for faculty development sessions on teaching professionalism
- discussion substrate for the clerkship dialogues on professionalism.

   The student narrative process within the STEP program has clearly been generative. The authentic stories students generate from their own experience have power, and this impact is amplified by the strong reactions others have when they hear or read these stories. The grounded narratives are truly having a *systemic* effect at IUSM and even outside our walls. How could this happen?

ORGANIZATIONAL CHANGE—A PREREQUISITE FOR IMPROVING EDUCATION FOR PROFESSIONALISM

Our IUSM initiative to foster professionalism by explicitly addressing and improving the informal curriculum has been guided by a new theory of human interaction called Complex Responsive Processes of Relating (CRPR) (Stacey, 2000). Integrating principles from complexity science, social constructionism, and relational psychology, this theory calls attention to the *self-organization* of patterns of meaning (ideas or themes) and patterns of relating (e.g., power relations, roles and etiquette) in the course of iterative communicative interactions. Exploring this theory in a bit more detail will permit a better understanding of how it has informed our activities at IUSM.

CRPR begins with G.H. Mead's insight that in the course of social interaction, meaning is created by the interactants, not merely exchanged. Using the example of one dog snarling at another, he points out that the ultimate meaning or significance of the gesture (the snarl) is plastic in the moment of its production—is it the initiation of a sequence of play, a ritualized display, a fight? Its meaning is completed only in the response that it elicits from the other dog. Stacey and his colleagues recognized in this interaction the signature form of a non-linear dynamic: 'A' influences and at the same time is influenced by 'B.' (This stands in contrast to a simple linear dynamic of 'A' causes 'B.') In the case of social interaction, the meaning of a gesture forms and is formed by the subsequent response. And the response is itself the next gesture in the sequence, forming and being formed by *its* response, and so on.

In the course of many iterations of this ongoing interaction of reciprocal influence, patterns will form, be sustained, and change, all in a spontaneous and self-organizing manner—that is, apart from the intentions of or direction by any participant. Two concrete examples from everyday experience may help make this clear.

The first example involves a conversation between two colleagues. At a lunch break from work in their laboratory, Dr. A makes a comment that Dr. B connects quite serendipitously with something she just read, prompting a new thought which she promptly shares with A. A grasps the new idea and takes it further and on they go. By the end of the back-and-forth exchange, A and B have created a new theory, a new organizational plan or some other transformative pattern of thinking. Neither A nor B embarked upon the conversation with the intention of creating something new; it just happened.

In the second example, Dr. B joins a pre-existing group—perhaps he has just accepted a new assignment to his school's curriculum committee. At his first meeting, he notices how others are behaving to discern what the norms are and quickly learns how to fit in. At the next meeting, another new person joins and observes B to learn how to fit in. After some period of time, the composition of the group could have turned over entirely—none of the original participants remaining—yet the pattern of interaction could continue unchanged. There are countless examples of cultural patterns (and sadly, patterns of intense conflict) that are self-propagating across hundreds of years. Again, no one directs or controls this process; it is self-organizing. These two examples illustrate three important properties of patterns in human interaction: they are self-organizing; capable of exhibiting remarkable continuity, even in the face of disturbances; and capable of being transformed unexpectedly by the rapid amplification of very small disturbances.

There are three further implications of the theory of CRPR to note before we return to our discussion of the informal curriculum and organizational culture change.   *First*, health care organizations, professional roles, reimbursement systems, and systems of knowledge about disease and treatment are all aspects of socially constructed reality. They represent patterns of thinking and relating that arise, persist and change in the course of iterative human interaction, as we have just described above. As self-organizing patterns, they are not subject to our designs or control. But they are subject to our influence, which leads to the second implication. *Second*, as human beings (unlike snarling dogs) we have the capacity to reflect on the continuous pattern-making in progress in each moment and in the case of patterns of continuity, to notice in what way our own behavior supports their propagation. Then, for patterns that we find undesirable, we can choose to participate in a different manner—to intentionally introduce a disturbance in the hope that it might propagate (but with no ability to predict or control what happens). So the practical implications of CRPR are to attend closely to here-and-now relational dynamics and be mindful of the way in which we are participating. The only means we have to introduce change is to change the nature of our own participation here in the living present, and the results we get will be unpredictable.

The *third* implication, and perhaps the most radical, is that our identities—the "personhood" associated with each physical body—is itself a pattern of meaning that is created, perpetuated and altered in the course of ongoing social interaction (Stacey, 2003). Our thinking is a private conversation of thoughts, subject to the same dynamics of iterative interactions, non-linear dynamic and emergent patterns of continuity and novelty that characterize conversations between people. Themes flow back and forth between social (interpersonal) and private (intrapersonal) conversations and it is in this fashion that ambient environmental patterns become incorporated into the self.

Returning to the story of our project to influence the informal curriculum at IUSM, we recognize that the informal curriculum or organizational culture at IUSM consists of self-organizing self-perpetuating patterns of relating that are being re-enacted in each moment, independent of anyone's intentions or control. Our only means of introducing change in these patterns is to change the nature of our own way of participating in them at each moment in the hope that others will then change as well. Each time we or anyone else steps outside a usual pattern, it constitutes a small disturbance that may or may not amplify and spread. The disturbances we have introduced tend to be relational; for example, inviting storytelling by students or at meetings where the conversation is typically analytic, or introducing practices such as describing something that has gone well since a previous meeting, or reflecting on what has been successful about a current meeting. . The use of *student stories* in a faculty development session or in a department's grand rounds is another form of disturbance. Introducing narrative—a more personal and subjective form of discourse—into these typically objective and analytic discussions establishes a new precedent and makes it more likely that stories will be shared again in the future. In some, but certainly not all cases, patterns like these are taking hold and have become the new norm for standing committees, curricula, management, and larger elements of the IUSM academic community.

The STEP Program is one part of a larger project at IUSM (the Relationship-Centered Care Initiative, RCCI) that is pursuing a shift in the culture of the organization to enhance our performance in the missions of our academic medical center—education, research, clinical care and service to the people of Indiana (Suchman et al., 2004). Perhaps the greatest "disruption" this larger project has created is to change the pattern of how people think about their own organization, to disturb that pattern of meaning called "organizational identity." Using the organizational change method of appreciative inquiry, we identified themes about the informal curriculum of

IUSM at its best by eliciting stories from students, faculty and staff, and then disseminated these themes in many venues. In this way, a more positive and hopeful image of the school is starting to form and a growing number of people are beginning to believe that change is really possible. We are also seeking to foster a new way of being together—a new pattern of relating— that consists of noticing and talking about relational process as it is happening (*"What's happening here right now?"*). This capacity liberates individuals and groups from automatically reproducing existing patterns and gives them the ability to explore and change their patterns mindfully, an organization-wide analogue to the mindfulness arising among students at IUSM of the professionalism behaviors all around them.

The whole RCCI project is in service of fostering professionalism at IUSM—a personal ethic and professional identity of self-awareness, empathy towards others and self, collaboration and shared decision-making. The idea that this could be accomplished by means of changing the social environment of medical educations rests on the assumption that themes in the environment can be internalized. CRPR shows how this is possible, as patterns of meaning from public (social conversation) are taken up in the private conversation of individuals.

PROFESSIONAL, PERSONAL, AND ORGANIZATIONAL DEVELOPMENT: A NEXUS

"The resident took care of a patient with bipolar disorder who was admitted for periorbital cellulitis and psychiatric medication noncompliance. The attending staff physician was unable to convince the patient to undergo treatment, but the resident was able to talk with the patient, calm her down, and show the patient the reasons she needed to be treated. The resident did this with such honesty and knowledge of both the patient's acute medical problem as well as her mental illness that she was able to connect with the patient when the attending staff physician was not able to. The patient ultimately received medical treatment and resumed her bipolar medications again. The level of care for this patient was impacted by the resident's compassion and patience to continue to try when the attending staff physician had had enough." The student checked: Excellence and Scholarship; Caring, Compassion, and Communication; Leadership; Knowledge and Skills.

You must be the change you want to see in the world.
Mahatma Gandhi

There are, of course, many ways to establish a wonderful environment for students of medicine to become the admirable professionals they hope to be. Most require time and resources—*lots* of time and *lots* of resources. The historical development of academic centers of excellence in medicine in the United States required closing many schools that failed to measure up to the German scientific medical education standard that was the benchmark a century ago. The biomedical revolution, the emergence of national accreditation, national examinations for certification and licensing, and the application of university-wide standards for academic excellence to schools of medicine all evolved from this starting point. Despite the development of rigorous objective standards, academic medical centers today still foster cynical attitudes among students of medicine towards the very field of work they seek to enter. We can do better, but improvement will require us to think explicitly about the knowledge, skills, and values we seek to promote. We must learn to be mindful of the personal, professional, and organizational environments we create in each moment, and find strategies to change ourselves, our workgroups, and our organizations in order to create greater alignment of our aspirations, our classroom teaching, and our own actions in the academic medical center environment.

We do not have lots of time and resources to do this work, given the high expectations and present need of our society for professionalism in medicine. There are ways and resources to succeed, and we hope this IUSM case report has illuminated one way forward. In the short run, it relies heavily on the courage of a few in an academic community to strike a spark and on the power of narrative to inform and motivate. Even within our large and complex organization, the informal curriculum—our day-to-day lives—and the formal curriculum can resonate with one another. Stories of the ordinary, especially narratives rooted in our deepest values, inspire us to action, shifting the center of gravity and culture of the organization. Our greatest challenge as a faculty of medicine may be to see ourselves as our students see us, to become mindful of the values we express through our actions and articulate about what we are trying to do and be. With the energy and inventiveness of IUSM faculty who have been inspired to take personal action by stories that "*remind them of why they got into medicine in the first place*," and with the authenticity of students (and their reinvigorated elders) who have their "feet on the ground and fresh eyes," a new culture of professionalism is being created and will be passed forward.

REFERENCES

Cruess, S.R., Johnston, S., & Cruess, R.L. (2004). Profession: A working definition for medical educators. *Teaching and Learning in Medicine, 16*, 74-76.

Freidson, E. (2001). *Professionalism: The third logic.* Chicago: The University of Chicago Press.

Hall, M.A., Dugan, E., Zheng, B., & Mishra, A.K. (2001). Trust in physicians and medical institutions: What is it, can it be measured, and does it matter? *Milbank Quarterly, 79*, 613-639.

Indiana University School of Medicine. (1996). The Indiana initiative: Physicians for the 21st century. Accessed from the website: http://meded.iusm.iu.edu/programs/comptmanual.pdf.

Inui T.S., (2003). *A flag in the wind: Educating for professionalism in medicine.* Washington, DC: Association of American Medical Colleges.

Inui T.S., (2004). Passion for the profession. *Indiana University Medicine, Winter*, 2-5.

Members of the Medical Professionalism Project (ABIM Foundation, ACP-ASIM Foundation, European Federation of Internal Medicine). (2002). Medical professionalism in the new millennium: A physician charter. *Annuals of Internal Medicine,136*, 243-246.

National Board of Medical Examiners (2004). Assessment of professional behaviors. *NBME Examiner, Spring/Summer*, 1-3. Accessed July 1, 2005 from the website: http://www.nbme.org/Examiners/SpringSummer2004/news.htm

Parsons, T. (1968). Professions. In D. L. Sills (Ed.), *International encyclopedia of the social sciences.* New York: Macmillan-Free Press.

Stacey, R. (2000). *Strategic management and organizational dynamics: The challenge of complexity*, 3rd edition. Harlow, England: Pearson Education, Ltd.

Stacey, R. (2003). *Complexity in group processes: A radically social understanding of individuals.* Hove, England: Brunner-Routledge.

Suchman, A.L., Williamson, P.R., Litzelman, D.K., Frankel, R.M., Mossbarger, D.L., & Inui, T.S. (2004). Towards an informal curriculum that teaches professionalism: Transforming the social environment of a medical school. *Journal of General Internal Medicine, 19*, 501-504.

Sullivan, W.M. (1995). *Work and integrity: The crisis and promise of professionalism in America.* New York: HarperCollins.

Testerman, J.K., Morton, K.R., Loo, L.K., Worthley, J.S., & Lamberton, H.H. (1996). The natural history of cynicism in physicians. *Academic Medicine, 71*, S43-45.

Chapter 10

THE PROBLEM WITH EVALUATING PROFESSIONALISM
The Case Against the Current Dogma

Mark Kuczewski
Loyola University, Stritch School of Medicine

There are moments when beliefs are so widely held that challenges are simply dismissed out of hand and those who hold them are easily vilified. For example, when a nation is on a march to war, the public sentiment may make it impossible to question the wisdom or morality of such a bellicose posture. Politically astute members of the opposition know better than to challenge the prevailing viewpoint. They simply sit down and shut up or try to position themselves such that they may plausibly deny they had actually supported the war when it results in disaster. But, they carefully avoid directly confronting the common wisdom sentiment prior to disaster. They understand that that to do so would lead to their marginalization and likely produce no good effect anyway as the momentum they wish to blunt is irreversible.

Of course, scholars and educators are not politicians. Truth is supposed to be more important than prestigious positions on committees and commissions or than receiving large amounts of grant funding. We should never hesitate to say things that fly in the face of the received wisdom when we suspect it is mistaken. However, the reality is that the message to "Sit down and shut up" is as strong in academia as anywhere else. In fact, because funding follows and reinforces the received wisdom, it is likely to be virtually impossible to challenge in any significant manner. Such is the dogma that is developing around the assessment of medical professionalism.

The desire to promote medical professionalism is noble, worthwhile, and necessary. It is important, even critical, at this moment in U.S. history that medicine undertake this effort in a serious and effective way. As is well-known, medicine as a profession is threatened by competing forces on all sides. Payers and regulators are making the work of physicians unbearably bureaucratic. The imperatives of technology and technique may be eclipsing the interpersonal aspects of healing. Excessive fears of litigation are undermining the trust between physicians and patients. And shrinking resources are threatening the social status physicians have long occupied in the United States. As these and other factors pummel medicine, professional organizations are tempted to become preoccupied with the financial and social well-being of physicians to the point that physicians come to be seen by the public as just one more special interest group looking out for itself. As a result, all efforts to marshal resources to promote professionalism in medicine are noble in intent and to be applauded.

Physicians must self-regulate their behavior, work to keep their patients safe and to provide them with high quality care, and to promote health policies that are in the interest of the public. All of this is necessary if medicine is to maintain the public confidence necessary to a profession and not simply become a job or a special interest group. But, such an agenda requires nothing short of the character development of most physicians. It requires that physicians be virtuous, i.e., they have characters that are habituated routinely to discern and pursue the good of their patients and society. How to produce this kind of practitioner is not easily known. And how to take to scale an educational program to develop the character of the large numbers of students in each medical school and hospital residency program is an even more daunting task. Of course, the very same problem of shrinking resources that may undermine the professionalism of physicians makes it difficult to develop new, resource-intensive educational programs. Thus, efforts to promote professionalism will be most well-received if they are easily standardizable, reproducible, and, of course, easily measured and documented.

The demand for simple and objective measures is, of course, ubiquitous in our age. The term "quality improvement" has become synonymous with "quality improvement measure." As a result, education systems at every level demand objective and eschew seemingly subjective or labor-intensive approaches to evaluation. The fear of subjective elements in evaluation is probably even more acute in regard to a new pedagogical arena such as professionalism. Efforts to teach virtue or inform character have been met with skepticism since the time of Socrates. It would seem that for professionalism to save medicine from the dire straits we've described, it would need to at least pass the same tests of scientific measurement that are demanded of other areas of quality improvement and educational practice.

Who can argue with such obvious requirements? To argue against them would seem to be, at best, to be unscientific and regressive and, at worst, to be against accountability. Of course, the truth is seldom so pure and simple.

What I believe is happening is that the desire for objective assessment is determining how medical education construes professionalism. That is, the modes of assessment that are seemingly most objective are measures that primarily "catch the bad guys." Checklists (i.e., scales) of behaviors, critical incident reports, and 360 assessments are all more likely to be able to document unacceptable behavior than to encourage positive actions by the students.

At the same time, the literature suggests that there is much that focuses on more positive approaches to professionalism, namely approaches that focus on professionalism as an opportunity to renew medicine as a vocation in the service of one's patients and society (Creuss, Creuss, & Johnston, 2000), that focus on fostering a sense of commitment to the public good through direct service to the underserved and advocating for social justice in health care (Eckenfels, 1997; Coulehan & Williams, 2000; Rothman, 2000; Kuczewski, Bading, Langbein, & Henry, 2003; Kuczewski et al. forthcoming), and by evaluation of the environment in which students are taught to be sure that it is the kind of place that limits the negative messages it informally sends students (Stern, 1998, 1998(a); Hundert, Hafferty & Christakis, 1996). In addition, some programs are attempting to provide an atmosphere of care through support group sessions. When these are coupled with efforts to also appreciate the patient's perspective, an atmosphere of "care and be cared for" may be generated (Gibson, Coldwell & Kicwit, 2000).

Of course, the latter attempts that focus on larger themes do not as easily translate into the generation of data that each and every student has achieved at least minimal competency on some measure of professionalism. Those approaches that provide such data usually focus on a minimal part of what we hope professionalism can provide. As a result, we run the risk that assessment will drive the way we define professionalism, and there is some preliminary data that support this fear (Eggly, Brennan, & Wiese-Rometsch, 2005). As a result, the noble motive of objective assessment may actually cause the new professionalism movement to fail medicine and fail society. It will fail medicine by failing to renew it as a calling that inspires physicians, as a return to a calling to serve patients and the public. It will fail society by continuing the tendency to de-professionalize medicine and continue the tendency toward "job-ification." It will increase the oversight of physician behavior, but in that way, make it little different from other jobs that are closely monitored. This will leave unfulfilled society's need for civic-minded leadership in health care.

WHAT IS PROFESSIONALISM? THE INCREDIBLE SHRINKING DOMAIN

One of the issues that immediately confronts any discussion of professionalism is simply the question of its definition. When one hears the word, it tends to stand for the opposite of whatever one's current pet peeve is. That is, it stands for reining in conflicts of interest when one is scandalized by the influence of pharmaceutical representatives, and it stands for candid and compassionate communication skills when one is frustrated by the lack of information the physician is providing. We legitimately could add to this list almost endlessly. Issues from reporting and peer review of medical error and physician impairment to advocacy for the uninsured all have claims to being a part of professionalism. Given this plethora of connotations, it is likely that there will never be one agreed-upon definition among all professional organizations and authors.

Nevertheless, most writers in this area find the duty to safeguard the interests of the patient as central to the notion of professionalism. This is sometimes expressed in terms of characteristics of the physician such as altruism and accountability that foster the best interests of the patient.

The terminology used to describe these qualities varies. Altruism, for example, may be unfortunate as it sounds somewhat saintly while professionalism connotes promoting the patient's good as being concordant with one's interests. But, for our present purposes, what is important to note is the broadness of the way professionalism tends to be construed in the vernacular. The only thing that seems to be excluded is the actual content of medical knowledge, yet a duty to be competent in one's medical knowledge is clearly entailed. This broad construal has been reflected in the influential work of the American Board of Internal Medicine's (ABIM) *Project Professionalism*, which resulted in the oft-quoted ABIM *Physician Charter* (Medical Professionalism Project, 2002).

I have made my own attempt to contribute to defining professionalism by characterizing it as "the norms that guide the relationships in which physicians engage in the care of patients" (Kuczewski et al., 2003, p. 161). This definition attempts to give primacy to the good of the patient as the measure and ordering principle of medical professionalism. It also emphasizes that promoting the good of the patient is dependent on successfully managing a number of other relationships such as those with other health-care team members, one's practice group and practice facilities, vendors, government, and ultimately with the general public.

For the purposes of evaluation, skills must be delineated in order to be assessed. Clearly the most influential force in this regard has been the Accreditation Council for Graduate Medical Education (ACGME), the organization that accredits residency programs. The ACGME divided residency education into six content domains: patient care, medical knowledge, practice-based learning and improvement, interpersonal and communication skills, professionalism, and systems-based practice. Their approach has been highly influential partly because of the thought, care, and diligence they have exercised in developing and implementing their outcomes project. In addition, because preparation for residency is the goal of medical education, the list has influenced medical educators across the country.

Two features of the ACGME approach are noteworthy for our purposes. First, what is most clearly considered professionalism is traditional medical ethics (e.g., informed consent, confidentiality, end-of-life care and the new area of cultural competence, with a nod toward business ethics through conflict of interest). As residency education is far more widespread than medical education and each program must meet its accreditation requirements, it is likely that professionalism will become more and more identified with medical ethics, flavored with cultural sensitivity.

But under the domain of professionalism, the ACGME also adds a somewhat vague outcome that residents are expected to "demonstrate respect, compassion, and integrity; a responsiveness to the needs of patients and society that supercedes self-interest; accountability to patients, society, and the profession; and a commitment to excellence and on-going professional development" (ACGME *Outcome Project*, 1999). This particular outcome seems to focus on clinical bearing including altruistic devotion to patients and to include accountability considerations. And its reference to society harkens back to the broader ABIM conception of professionalism. However, unless this outcome is given concrete content that must be evaluated by ACGME auditors, few programs will identify professionalism with this broader connotation.

As a result, the second important feature of the ACGME approach concerns what is not considered the focal meaning of professionalism. Namely, considerations of how the health-care system works have gone mainly into their own area of competence, i.e., systems-based practice, and other relationship issues such as working with team members and communicating well with patients have similarly been assigned to other domains.

I do not intend to criticize the recent work of the ACGME as it has been a landmark in the history of professional education. However, we must note how what they have outlined as professionalism may be conceived so narrowly that it threatens to deprive the term of its most promising aspects while adding the negative (albeit necessary) connotation of accountability. Of course, definitions and lists of outcomes are merely definitions and lists, not practices. In many educational initiatives, e.g., a course on the business and justice aspects of medicine, the problem of what falls under which competence is artificial as the initiative will likely attend to outcomes from multiple domains such as professionalism and systems-based practice. But if one sets out to build assessments for each domain, the most likely thing one would do to assess professionalism would be to make sure there was a system in place to hold students accountable for their behavior. That is, there would be reliable ways of documenting negative behaviors such as violations of confidentiality or disrespecting of patients or superiors; one might also add an exercise that tests for traditional bedside ethics skills such as "breaking bad news" to a patient.

While delineating these skills and documenting assessment of them is commendable, it potentially helps to set the stage for the downfall of the professionalism movement. That is it takes all the fun out of professionalism while stashing the policing aspects under this label. Thus, the hope for the rhetoric of professionalism to re-inspire a radical return to the vocation of medicine and to a calling to serve society can be hindered in this conceptualization.

But this conceptual framework is likely to be only a small factor in undermining the new professionalism. Despite this list of domains, the vernacular use of professionalism as stand in for the broad array of communication, ethical, legal, and social aspects of medical practice is unlikely to be obliterated easily. Of far greater danger are the inherent biases in the way we approach assessment.

ASSESSING PROFESSIONALISM: THE STATE OF THE PRACTICE

Objectivity in the educational assessment of student performance is certainly a desirable thing. Medical students and residents are busy trying to hone their clinical knowledge and skills and to become like their mentors. A new curricular area that requires their time and attention is likely to be met with initial skepticism. The addition to the curriculum will fare better if its subject matter is well-defined, the learning objectives articulated, and the assessment perceived as objective and fair. This is especially true when the subject matter is from the "softer" side of medicine. Unfortunately, such hopes may be a bit too much to require of a professionalism curriculum and we might have to be content to follow Aristotle's lead in asking as much precision as the subject matter allows (Aristotle, *NE* I.3 1094b13-14).

In the most comprehensive review of assessment methods of professionalism to date, Louise Arnold states, "No single method exists for the reliable and valid evaluation of professional behavior" (Arnold, 2002, p. 507). However, she does not despair of this task but argues that the array of assessment tools is "rich" but that "their measurement properties should be strengthened" (Arnold, 2002, p. 503). However, in her reviews of several of the most common assessment techniques, one cannot help but become concerned for several reasons. First, many of the approaches seen as most promising tend to help educators document the poor or offensive behavior of students and residents or assess fairly small or trivial behaviors. Second, when implementing these promising methods, the requirements of the learning environment are likely to substitute *volume* of documentation for *meaningful* observation. Third, these approaches will, therefore, lead to cynicism and disdain for attempts to introduce professionalism into the curriculum unless these approaches are seen as being part of a larger and more meaningful context. Let us look at each of these concerns in more detail.

The most obvious way to evaluate professionalism would seem to be to observe a professional or unprofessional behavior and document it. As a result, devising scales that list qualities or behaviors for raters to check off or score would seem helpful (Phelan, Obenshain & Galey, 1993; Ginsburg et al., 2000). This is analogous to a list of clinical procedures a student might have to perform in front of an instructor. Unfortunately, the parallel breaks down quickly. Interacting respectfully and effectively with team members, being prompt and courteous, and other routine professional behaviors would not seem to be meaningfully assessed by observing a single instance of the behavior as a procedure might. As a result, the tendency is to allow a student to go through a rotation and then make the assessment. But, as observation of students by a clerkship or program director is sporadic and he or she will find it difficult to recall relevant instances of these professional behaviors of each student or resident, the grader will find it easiest to pass the candidate unless an incident of unsatisfactory behavior has been noticed. Being deemed professional is simply the absence of having been unprofessional.

When using such scales, being professional will not only be considered the norm but will thereby be equated with all routine behavior. Only negative, unprofessional behavior will actually "count" in the sense of actually being assessed. This trivializes professional behavior. It follows that the assessment system would be more direct and transparent if it simply made targeting unprofessional behavior the goal. As a result, critical incident reporting systems would seem commendable at first glance (Papadakis, Osborn, Cooke, & Healy, 1999). Such systems provide documentation of negative behavior and provide an opportunity for feedback. The documentation may also be helpful in dismissing chronic offenders. Of course, one must be careful that the system is calibrated so as to be fair, e.g., major offenses are met with stronger responses than are small or inconsequential ones. However, having a critical incident system likely means that many small trivial behaviors will be documented or that some small incidents will create a negative halo effect. As small transgressions are more common than large ones, the typical critical incident report will document a small offense that might seem to be nit-picking to the student or resident.

Second, it is easy to see how volume will come to replace significance. While clerkship or program directors have limited access to each person he or she must grade, there are many other persons in the clinical setting who can be recruited to provide feedback to the student or resident. Having similar rating scales or reports completed by peers, nurses, or virtually anyone who interacts with the medical student or resident, could provide greater insight into how one participates as a member of a team or care giver. When one collects such evidence from the circle of persons with whom the student interacts, it is called a 360 degree evaluation. To be clear, it is important that students learn to be members of health-care teams. And, we know that other members of the team may see the student's performance differently from the student's superiors. But the net effect of multiple checklists repeatedly being filled out about a student will likely result in even more documentation of small transgressions.

As the volume of documentation of small transgressions grows, it furthers the possibility that professionalism will come to be seen as surveillance of the trivial. The result may be that these approaches will lead to cynicism and disdain for attempts to introduce professionalism into the curriculum. However, we cannot entirely forgo the effort to document and remediate unprofessional behavior. Some efforts in this direction are warranted because part of what the public expects from the profession of medicine is peer review and correction of unprofessional behavior. However, as physicians face increasing regulatory, compliance, and interpersonal demands, simply adding one more set of cumbersome demands within medical and residency education, a set that is generally relatively minor most of the time, is likely to only add to the frustration and cynicism of the assessors and the assessed unless these approaches are seen as being part of a larger and more meaningful context.

What I fear is that the result of these standard assessment methods will be that medicine de-values rather than values professionalism. Because the connotations and denotations that accompany professionalism in these assessments seem small and negative, they hold little chance of revitalizing the practitioners' commitment to medicine. As a result, advocating for the proliferation of these approaches and attempting to make them more objective, valid, verifiable, reproducible, and scientific simply misses the point and possibly makes the problem worse. We should advocate that our medical and medical education institutions focus on helping medical students, residents, and faculty to value professionalism rather than objectively assess it.

VALUING PROFESSIONALISM: ASSESSING THE ENVIRONMENT, CARING FOR STUDENTS, PROMOTING JUSTICE

Valuing and evaluating professionalism seem to have become equated. But, as we have seen, methods of evaluation are often chosen for reasons inherent to the evaluation process, e.g., the seeming "scientific" or "objective" nature of the method, the ease of use of the method, and/or the tangible nature of the outcome of using the method. But, as I have suggested, such methodological virtues may be illusory. At best, they may lead to one-dimensional evaluation in which negative behaviors are documented in order to be remediated. At worst, much effort is expended to produce shallow or illusory assessment of learners with the result that the very term professionalism comes to be viewed with cynicism or disdain. Obviously, this would be a tragic outcome given the hopes for the new professionalism movement. What could be done differently?

When evaluation methods focus only on negative behaviors or become more form than substance, professionalism is de-valued in the eyes of the participants. The obvious remedy would be to begin by asking "How can a school or training environment demonstrate that professionalism is valued there?" Notice how a shift from evaluation to valuing changes the emphasis from the student to the environment. In fact, it is hard to understand how such a question ever resulted in the current array of evaluative techniques. The missing link is the current centrality of the concept of competency.

While the current emphasis on competencies has much to commend it, it also has an inherent weakness. Namely, when the goal is to assess competencies, we immediately seek a method to evaluate each and every learner and we must set the minimum level of competence that each learner must demonstrate to be considered competent. The emphasis is on the lowest common denominator of proficiency (sometimes defined as the absence of an incident of incompetence) and the task becomes documentation of the evaluation of each and every learner according to this minimum measure. But if we don't start with the assumption of the competency approach, we might end in measures that evaluate the environment in terms of its likelihood to produce physicians who value professionalism. That is, we should assess how the environment demonstrates that it values professionalism.

Of course, an attempt to evaluate an environment comes with its own epistemological and pedagogical assumptions. These reasonable assumptions, where X = professionalism, include:

1. If we identify, highlight, and reinforce instances of value X, then X is more likely to recur.
2. If we support students cognitively and affectively when value X is threatened, value X is more likely to withstand the threat.
3. Value X will likely be internalized over time and become a part of the reflective and behavioral repertoire of the learner.

These foundational assumptions are, indeed, assumptions but they are similar to those that undergird any approach to teaching and learning. That is, we are simply assuming that an environment that places what it wants in the spotlight and rewards and supports learners who emulate the desired behaviors will produce the desired learning. It might not produce it in each and every learner to the same extent. It will, however, likely achieve higher overall levels of the behavior(s).

From the time of Socrates, Plato, and Aristotle, teaching virtue has been about looking to the paradigmatic instances of virtues and persons who exemplify the virtues. The good person is the measure of excellence, not the person who merely avoids vice. In some ways, we are simply calling attention to the importance of role modeling. However, I am also suggesting that by focusing on positive instances and reinforcing them, we may strongly influence the educational environment and produce effective cultural change. When the environment values professionalism, those who train within it will achieve higher levels of professionalism.

How should we demonstrate that we value professionalism in the medical school and clinical environments? There is no one set of answers. But the following strongly suggest themselves.

First, the most highly regarded clinicians and administrators must be involved in the teaching of professionalism. Whatever aspect of professionalism we are talking about, from clinical teamwork to social justice, it is important that teaching this aspect include and involve deans, department chairs, program directors, and faculty and administrators who are perceived as accomplished. Again, role modeling is the most effective tool in fostering virtue. Sending a "B-team" of ethicists will be effective with some students but will send a message that professionalism is not important in the "real world" of clinical medicine. But, a multidisciplinary group that integrates ethicists and policy experts with clinicians and administrators sends the opposite message, i.e., that professionalism is multi-faceted and worthy of exploration.

Second, students must have an opportunity to reflect on their formative experiences related to professionalism and receive feedback. Medical training is fast-paced and packed with a variety of potent experiences. Furthermore, many students participate in a wide variety of extracurricular activities including service learning, research of various kinds, and professional associations. These experiences will be formative, positively or negatively, whether students get to reflect on them or not. But, student reflection on these experiences is likely to be helpful in two ways. First, reflection enables the student to directly confront his or her affective responses to persons and situations and to try to integrate them into a larger perspective. Second, reflection may enable a student to inventory his or her strengths and areas in need of improvement and to generate a plan to utilize strengths and improve upon deficiencies. Some structured approach to reflection such as a mentored portfolio experience or discussion group can facilitate such reflection.

Mentorship or discussion partners can be an important aspect of the reflective experience. Others can relate to the student's thoughts and feelings, reinforce the student's positive responses, and help to re-direct the student when particular experiences have skewed or distorted the student's perspective (Kuczewski, et al., forthcoming). Such partners in reflection reinforce the importance of professional development and can create a supportive community. We would ultimately hope that such mentoring and peer feedback would ultimately help to develop the student's self-assessment skills. Such self-assessment is typically decried as unreliable (Ginsburg et al., 2000; Arnold 2002), but few interventions to improve them have been created or explored.

Third, students who are high achievers in professionalism should receive public recognition. That is, many students do a wide variety of things we see as relevant to the development of professionalism. Many provide significant service to the underserved, provide leadership to important student organizations, and excel in relevant parts of the required curriculum. Such excellence should be routinely identified and honored in high-profile venues. It is important that all such honorings stress that this aspect of medicine, i.e., professionalism, is an area in which all can achieve similar excellence and honor with sufficient effort. It must not reinforce stereotypes that this area is the province of a small number of altruistic and saintly persons. As a result, honors programs in professionalism or medical humanism should be effort- and performance-based rather than limited to a restricted group chosen by reputation.

Fourth, institutions must seek to stamp out the negative behaviors in the powerful, not just the powerless. While I hope to refocus us on the positive rather than the negative aspects of professionalism, students will find even the most service- and justice-oriented institution disingenuous if all negative behaviors by attending physicians are tolerated. Thus, while the development of "professionalism police" may be unwelcome, some effort to routinely assess the negative behavior and hidden curriculum within an institution and to promote improvement of that environment is necessary. Fortunately, instruments to assess the environment are available (Arnold, Blank, & Cipparrone, 1998).

Finally, valuing professionalism will mean a return to defining it broadly and fostering attention to more than the negative aspects. Being a professional must be about a recommitment to the roots of medicine, to regaining its status as the healing profession, and to aiding physicians in recovering their calling. As the new professionalism has arisen partly from the frustration of physicians who feel buffeted about by the current practice climate, the new professionalism must look to ways to help physicians provide leadership to change the environment. This will mean that the agenda for the professionalism movement must include societal and health system aspects as well as an aspect devoted to the physician-patient relationship. If medicine is to regain the public trust by advocating for the public good as well as making the system more humane and less bureaucratic, professionalism efforts must include these focuses.

A curriculum that values professionalism in the full sense will include courses on medical economics, health systems, public health including health disparities, and social justice. Similarly, departmental grand rounds, named lectures, and continuing medical education offerings will focus on these topics and consider them from a macro- and micro-economic perspective. Physicians at all levels will feel that "real" doctors concern themselves with financing and delivery systems to simplify the access issues and promote the health of our citizenry, and not expect that their associations will focus only their own malpractice premiums or reimbursement rates (Creuss & Creuss, 1997).

At the same time, the "healer" aspects of professionalism must not be forgotten (Creuss, Creuss, & Johnston, 2000). It has become a commonplace that as technology has become more advanced and medicine more effective, the world of the doctor and patient has become increasingly quiet. The revival of medical humanities that pre-dated the professionalism movement sought to remedy this through fostering appreciation for the patient's perspective (Arnold, 2002). This approach has been supplemented by the techniques of quality improvement and evidence-based medicine in an effort to foster the physician's communication skills and approaches to such matters as end-of-life decision-making and pain management. In essence, the aspects of professionalism, i.e., medical ethics, that are placed front and center in the ACGME elaboration of competency in professionalism, must also be furthered.

We must not fall into the trap of thinking that the latter comprises a group of settled issues and proven pedagogical techniques. Despite a fair amount of attention to this area, issues concerning physician-patient communication around end-of-life such as unilateral DNR policies (i.e., futility) remain hotly contested. Furthermore, while large programs have sprung up to teach better end-of-life care, these tend to work on fairly static models in which the "bad news" is clear and all physicians have to do is learn to break it to patients. There is still much to be understood about negotiating care for patients who suffer from long-term chronic illnesses that will eventually prove fatal (Shugarman, Lorenz, & Lynn, 2005).

Finally, while the medical humanities have come under fire for the lack of evidence of the efficacy of techniques (Kao & Reenan, 2005) we must not abandon the hope that a renewed interest in the medical humanities and professionalism can eventually provide us with better way to help physicians understand themselves, their patients, and the communities they serve (Kuczewski, 2004).

REFERENCES

Accreditation Council for Graduate Medical Education (ACGME). (1999). *Outcomes project*. Retrieved July 11, 2005 from the website: http://www.acgme.org/outcome/comp/compFull.asp
Aristotle. (1999). *Nicomachean ethics*. (T. Irwin, Trans.). New York: Hackett Publishing Company.

Arnold, E.L., Blank, L.L., Race, K.E., & Cipparrone, N. (1998). Can professionalism be measured? The development of a scale for use in the medical education environment. *Academic Medicine, 73*, 1119-1121.

Arnold, L. (2002). Assessing professional behavior: Yesterday, today, and tomorrow. *Academic Medicine, 77*(6), 502-515.

Coulehan, J., & Williams, P. (2000). Professional ethics and social activism: Where have we been? Where are we going? In D. Wear & J. Bickel (Eds.), *Educating for professionalism: Creating a culture of humanism in medical education.* Iowa City: University of Iowa Press.

Creuss, R.L., & Creuss, S.R. (1997). Teaching medicine in the service of healing. *Academic Medicine, 72*, 941-952.

Creuss, R.L., Creuss, S.R., & Johnston, S.E. (2000). Professionalism and medicine's social contract. *Journal of Bone Joint Surgery, 82A*, 1189-1194.

Eckenfels, E.J. (1997). Contemporary medical students' quest for self-fulfillment through community service. *Academic Medicine, 72*, 1043-1050.

Eggly, S., Brennan, S., & Wiese-Rometsch, R. (2005). Once when I was on call. . . Theory versus reality in training for professionalism. *Academic Medicine, 80*(4), 371-375.

Gibson, D.D., Coldwell, L.L., & Kiewit, S.F. (2000). Creating a culture of professionalism. *Academic Medicine, 75*, 509.

Ginsburg, S., Regehr, G., Hatala, McNaughton, N., Frohna, A., Hodges, B., et. al. (2000). Context, conflict, and resolution: A new conceptual framework for evaluating professionalism. *Academic Medicine, 75*(10), S6-S11.

Hundert, E.M., Hafferty, F., & Christakis, D. (1996). Characteristics of the informal curriculum and trainees' ethical choices. *Academic Medicine, 71*(6), 624-642.

Kao, A., & Reenan, J. Wit is not enough. In this volume.

Kuczewski, M.G., Villaume, F., Chang, H., Fitz, M., Bading, E., & Michelfelder, A. (in press). Can justice be taught? Valuing justice and professionalism in the medical school curriculum. In K. Parsi & M. Sheehan (Eds.), *Healing as vocation: A primer on professionalism,* Washington, DC: Rowman & Littlefield.

Kuczewski, M.G., Bading, E., Langbein, M., & Henry, B. (2003). Fostering professionalism: The Loyola model. *Cambridge Quarterly of Healthcare Ethics, 12*(2), 161-166.

Kuczewski, M.G. (2004). Re-reading *On Death and Dying:* What Elisabeth Kubler-Ross can teach clinical bioethics. *American Journal of Bioethics, 4*(4), W19-W23.

Medical Professionalism Project. (2002). Medical professionalism in the new millennium: A physician charter. *Annals of Internal Medicine, 136*, 243-246.

Papadakis, M.A., Osborn, E.H.S., Cooke, M., & Healy, K. (1999). A strategy for detection and evaluation of unprofessional behavior in medical students. *Academic Medicine, 74*, 980-990.

Phelan, S., Obenshain, S.S., & Galey,W.R. (1993). Evaluation of the non-cognitive professional traits of medical students. *Academic Medicine, 68*(10), 799-803.

Rothman, D.J. (2000). Medical professionalism – focusing on the real issues. *New England Journal of Medicine, 342*, 1284 -1286.

Shugarman, L.R., Lorenz, K., & Lynn, J. (2005). End-of-life care: An agenda for policy improvement. *Clinics in Geriatric Medicine, 21*(1), 255-272.

Stern, D.T. (1998). In search of the informal curriculum: When and where professional values are taught. *Academic Medicine, 73*(10), S28-S30.

Stern, D.T. (1998a) Practicing what we preach? An analysis of the curriculum of values in medical education. *American Journal of Medicine, 104*, 569-575.

Chapter 11

HOW MEDICAL TRAINING MANGLES PROFESSIONALISM
The Prolonged Death of Compassion

Cynthia A. Brincat
University of Michigan

I am a philosopher by training and a physician by vocation. What this means is that my sensibilities are profoundly practical, but I can take more time than anyone else to explain and defend them. Starting my academic career as a junior faculty member in various academic departments, I have become especially attuned to pedagogical approaches and administrative demands as well as the overt politics of one academy as compared to another. Moving from the humanities to medicine, I have found that the more things change, the more they stay the same. That is, the trends appearing in one department are likewise made manifest in another. Easing out of higher education to go to medical school, I left behind cries for professional responsibility across the curriculum, and applied ethicists including myself working to figure out a way to meet that demand. In medicine the same cries are at play—doctors need to be astute professionals—and many are working to address that need at various levels of medical education and practice. Not only are we working to address these needs, but we are continuously faced with proving how we have addressed them as outcomes assessment is more and more the vogue.

Transitioning from a teaching professional to a medical professional, the demands for professionalism from a moral perspective are just as important, but practically seem more so. This is true because of the fact that, when our professionalism in medicine fails, the stakes are high insofar as it really can be a matter of life or death. The vulnerability of illness and its far-reaching devastation is the consummate vulnerability of our own mortality, against which we are ultimately and eventually powerless. Against this backdrop, the present push for outcomes assessment has arisen. Somehow, when so much is at stake, we need to be certain our attempts at appropriately grounding professionalism are working. Or else, administrators need somehow to justify the present academic flavor of the day. Either way, through all of our attentions, the professionalism discourse in medicine has portrayed professionalism as if it were a patient at the end of life, near death by all of its machinations, as if something needs to be done at breakneck speed before the crisis is beyond salvation.

Rather than think of professionalism and its teaching as near death, the metaphor of futility is more appropriate. Thinking of professionalism via this framework is unusual, albeit apt. The same issues of end of life care are present here. Some are calling for more treatment, while others are seeking an end to treatment. People are just as convinced that without the treatment, the patient-professionalism will be lost. Or, if the treatment doesn't stop, the patient will lose all dignity. Like most things, the truth is somewhere in the middle, which is why the metaphor of futility works. Professionalism is ventilated, on tube feeds and without brain stem activity. Even so, we are hurling resources at it in such a manner that reflects a desperate and misplaced hope, however sincere, for a miracle. Professionalism, or at least pedagogy in professionalism, is limping along at the comparable cost of an ICU bed. Although the relationship of health care professionals to professionalism is not that of a disease that needs to be "cured," we are treating it as such as more and more interventions divorce it from compassion, its deepest root and spring. If we can slowly disconnect our machines, turn off our monitors, we can let professionalism in its present guise die. In its place, we can return to the values that drive professionalism and an approach to professionalism that cultivates its mainspring of compassion.

The professionalism crisis in medicine is, in many ways, manufactured. Most health care providers are true professionals as they do what they do not only with technical acumen but also with sensitivity to their greater social role. They care for their patients, bill appropriately and take their responsibilities as educators seriously. They love medicine and from that love or at least commitment springs a sense of responsibility. Alas, what of the others? Where do they come from and what do we do with them?

Here we are not thinking of those that prey on residents or medical students, commit billing fraud and abuse patients. The law and medical administrators take care of these egregious offenders eventually and no professionalism training in the world will ever address their lack of moral or even legal sensibilities. One can only hope that there are enough safeguards in the system to derail these individuals before they cause too much damage.

Instead, what about those somewhere in the middle? What of those that pad their billing, don't answer their pages, ignore medical students, abuse residents, and do these things only on the days when they have fought with their partner, gone too long without sleep or missed their second or third cup of coffee? It is these individuals that professional training seeks to change, prevent from forming or at least annoy once they are formed.

In what follows, I'll look at the manner in which our appropriate concern with moral mediocrity got swept away into an obsession with professionalism.

THE OBSESSION WITH PROFESSIONALISM

Medical education, training and supervision have become obsessed with professionalism, and they are doing so with a micro-management, sub-specialty style. That is, in medical training, we have attempted to articulate very specifically what is professional behavior. Consequently, as individuals move through their training, they are met with discord as it is, as if professionalism is re-invented depending upon whether one is at a pre-clinical, clinical, or house staff level. In critically assessing this discourse of discord, we would be well served to find its common underpinnings, and from there let our professional discourse begin. Until then, the professionalism discourse mimics that of its futility counterpart insofar as the patient isn't dying, but it certainly isn't being helped. At each level of medical training, the approach to professionalism is like that of multiple sub-specialists hovering over the patient, each intent on its own organ system, without concern for the whole. In breaking through the sub-specialist's discourse in the futility debate and breaking through the professionalism discourse in medical care, we come in contact with the patient, and thus get in touch with what makes caring manifest, which is compassion.

The discourse of professionalism did not appear *de novo* in the guise of mandates from the Accreditation Council for Graduate Medical Education or the Association of American Medical Colleges. Instead it came out of the dearth of professional vision in medicine and the ensuing crisis that came to a head in the 1970s. We can think of the situation as the overweight middle-aged hypertensive who decides it's a good idea to shovel the snow out of his driveway. Things were moving along well enough, but when the system was stressed, his coronary arteries couldn't hold up. Once the initial vulnerability hit, Paul Starr (1982) describes how outside forces were able to move into a void and thereby impact medicine's professional image, as a consequence of "the contradictions of accommodation and the generalization of rights." At first, players in medicine, or payers in medicine, were seen to have competing interests. That is, the practice of medicine was no longer about a health care provider and the service provided to a patient; instead it was about the provider, the patient and the person paying for that service. Furthermore, each of these players was having interests competing against one another. Consequently, groups of payers, the insurance industry, the employers and the government all sought to reform medicine and medical practice, and medicine as a profession became the all too willing victim of its own reform (Starr, 1982).

While those paying for health care were making demands on the way medicine as a profession should look, those receiving health care were making demands on the profession as well. In the crisis of the 1970s, health care was seen as a right against the backdrop of a system that had for the most part treated it as a privilege. At the same time, patients were realizing that in receiving the right of health care they too had rights such as informed consent, a freedom from paternalism and an ability to play a part in the decisions affecting them. While medicine had previously been practiced without such a great need for discussion of risks, benefits, alternatives and second opinions, it now had to redefine itself as it interacted with patients in a different manner. Some of this took place as a part of greater social reforms, such as the civil rights and the feminist movements, but much of it also took place as a consequence of a societal unwillingness to accept authority without question, just because it wanted to be accepted or had traditionally been accepted.

Rather than become organized or affiliated with the patient or even amongst themselves, physicians fell prey to intervention. Intervention took the form of regulations of care and cost, regulation to safeguard patient rights, and measures to redistribute resources. Of course this was not all bad, and many needed safeguards were put into place. But as more and more voices formed the discourse of the profession of medicine, likewise was formed the discourse of medical professionalism.

For our purposes, within the context of these new voices, medical education began to speak formally to the need for professional education, education not left up to the professionals themselves and not done by the professionals within the profession. So it was that education in professionalism was removed from the ability of one more experienced physician to teach the physician in training. A need was now seen to involve other points of view, those of ethicists, sociologists, historians and the like. Just as in its practice, in its professional image and the manner in which this was enacted in and of itself and to those in training, medicine was having to contend with being defined by outside forces (Starr, 1982).

As medicine lost control of its own image of itself as a profession and thus its own image of professionalism, it lost control of the *creation* of these images as different forces exerted their controls at each level of training and practice and various theorists and practitioners sought to define medical professionalism. In its various forms, the discussion at play can be seen as a reflection of the concerns of the multiple communities framing the discourse; that is, medical historians, sociologists and ethicists all have their own approach to framing the professionalism discourse. Yet as we transition from the control of one community to another, those framing the discourse change and in doing so the discourse itself changes. Consequently, the professionalism training of one level of medical training moves onto the next and the previous level is either met with discord, irrelevance or superceded. This is the case as medical students move from the pre-clinical to the clinical years and residents and fellows move to attending positions.

Although the need for external controls and professionalism education in medicine was well placed, it came at the cost of a faulty yet coherent discourse on professionalism and consequently a coherent professional identity. The previous discourse and identity however flawed was holistic, and in its absence, medical professionalism is schizophrenically defined by the outside forces that impact its formation. In what follows, we can see the various manifestations of professionalism in medical training and the discord that follows as trainees advance. Finally, we can look at from whence this discourse, regardless of its origin, springs. In doing so, medicine can reclaim professionalism as it reclaims its assumed previous motivation with a symbiotic relationship to its detractors that have filled the void and return to that which makes it meaningful—compassion.

PROFESSIONALISM IN MEDICAL TRAINING MADE MANIFEST

The pre-clinical years

The role of compassion is obviously central to my commentary. Implicitly, compassion is that value behind our professional action. It is the core of relational sensitivity that is central to medicine. Elsewhere medical professionalism has been defined in terms of obligation, and truly this responsibility is key. But there is something about the absolute revelation of illness in its vulnerability and the trust implicit in stewardship of someone's health that moves beyond this. When someone who is ill requires something of you and you respond, regardless of how tired you are, how many hassles you have dealt with, and how inconsequential your actions may be, that response comes about as a response between two people, not between a theory and its application, but in a moment of humanity that I am asserting as central to the relational sensitivity required of a medical professional. When professional discourse moves too far away from that, all is lost. Likewise, when medical professionalism is trusted to rely solely on this value without safeguards or grounding, we are no better. A balance between the two would be the ideal.

Yet, in the beginning of medical training, the images of the profession that appear most strongly are those tied to the symbols of the profession: the white coat, the stethoscope, the name badge and the like. Much of this becomes concrete with the white coat ceremony. As a first year student, you receive your white coat, often courtesy of the alumni association, and so it is that one doctor hands over "the mantle" to the next generation. This ceremonial sense of doctoring is short lived, and usually takes place in a classroom, where shortly thereafter the real work of the first two years of medical school begins, for the most part, divorced from patient contact. In that divorce lies a missed opportunity to maintain the motivation to keep relevant the chemical and biological theorems and the why of their importance.

The first years of medical school involve an immersion in first the function and then the dysfunction of the human system. With the amount of information coming at you, it is like taking a drink of water from a fire hose. Here begins the first training in medical professionalism. In most medical schools this takes the form of the obvious: don't lie, cheat or steal, show up on time and don't talk during lectures. The most patient interaction this involves is how to take a good history, with specific attention to difficult topics like sexual history, drug use and the like. Unfortunately, in most instances these histories take place between two medical students, one interviewing another in a role-playing exercise. Occasionally, in a diminishing number of medical schools, these interviews take place between a standardized patient and a medical student. Rarely in these first years of medical training do you experience the difficult reality of responding to a real human being dealing with his or her own health or its lack. Even with standardized patient, in their scripted presence, the interaction becomes yet another graded performance. Rarely do you have the real patient interaction such that you are the tenth person that day to ask someone if they have any drug allergies, to only get your head bitten off because they are tired of waiting to be seen, understood, examined or whatever, and they just want some relief and they can't understand why we have to ask the same things over and over again.

Thus, the first slight contact with patients is mediated by the construct of chief complaints, history of present illnesses and past medical and surgical histories. Patient contact, before it even substantively takes place, is mediated by a protection that is two-fold. First, during your pre-clinical years you rarely see patients, and second, when you do, it is thoroughly controlled. Moments that could be personally illustrative end up being removed from any meaningful context since the first year student is so focused on a process of data gathering rather than the person whose story is being gathered. This early training is described as setting up the dichotomy between what is to be held as true knowledge in contrast to what is to be considered as a subjective data point. So it is that the metabolic process of keto-acidosis is real, while the reason the teenager never got his insulin prescription refilled is deemed irrelevant.

As time and training progress, one sees enough of those teenagers in near comas, without transportation, with the adults in their lives working several jobs, so there is no one to get them to the pharmacy. Then the subjective story of the disease becomes as relevant as any lab value, because that is the basis and cause of the disease just as much as is a lack of endogenous insulin. But this relevance will not matter when the focus is merely on the disease process, divorced from the person to whom it belongs (Wear & Castellani, 2000).

So it is that anything to do with anything but science is disregarded and so disregarded are theoretical discussions of professionalism. The aspects of the curriculum tempered by outside forces—the sociologist, the philosophers and the historians who teach your "ethics" or "professionalism" courses— are bracketed as being just as irrelevant as a lack of transportation. This is not a new issue, and has been pointed to as occurring more obviously in the later clinical years of medical training. But here, already the roots of the discord are there as a consequence of the meat of professionalism, how we do what we do being divorced from the relational sensitivity that makes learning to do what we do well matter.

How to resolve the difficulties of those first two years is troubling. The difficulty lies in the lack of opportunity to come face to face with patients, for it is in that context that not only the profession of medicine but also medical professionalism is made meaningful. Without that context, amidst science bereft of humanity, your professional identity will seem nonsensical. Likewise, if the tools for you to make your professionalism discourse real are not grounded in real patient contact, they will likewise seem irrelevant. What would a solution to this dichotomy look like? The pre-clinical years, instead of teaching the rudimentary obvious lessons of the kindergarten playground could, with the help of the "outside" experts, begin to give pre-clinical trainees the tools to understand "the social, economic, and often messy political climates of health care systems and how such factors will directly influence the ways trainees will perform their life's work"(Wear & Castellani, 2000). This would involve a new conception of what is valuable in medical learning in the pre-clinical years, requiring a new basic education, which is taught *and* tested well. This testing would involve not only examinations, but also interaction with real patients, with opportunities to reflect on the grounding of our approaches as well as their application.

In short, since professionalism can't be understood divorced from a professional context, in these pre-clinical years medical student education has only two alternatives, or some sort of a combination thereof. It can deal with patients in a limited, safe context, taking histories, repeating physicals following on rounds with mouths shut and professional judgment turned off. Or students could be given the tools to cultivate a sense of professionalism via hearing the stories of other professionals, patients and families so that when students are faced with the issues that will inevitably arise, they may not have answers but at least they will be able to formulate the inescapable troubling questions and have had enough motivating patient contact to keep working at those questions.

The clinical years

Medical students typically enter into their clinical years understanding what makes up a good history and the steps of a broad physical exam. At best, they have been introduced to rudimentary language of moral maneuverings such as autonomy, beneficence, non-maleficence and justice, the universal script of principlism sans personhood (Beauchamp, 1994). The conflicts of clinical training aren't easily placed into these rubrics as they encompass not only patient-professional relationships but the relationships between professionals at varying levels from student to resident to attending to ancillary staff. In the rare instances where students have been given an idea of the greater issues at work in the discourse of medical professionalism, they have even more rarely been given an idea of what the issues might look like when addressed at their level of medical engagement. Medical students don't actually grapple with end of life care, allocation of scarce resources or even the disparity of health care. That is, curricular topics in professionalism rarely address the conflicts of the lowest rung of the ladder, let alone the tarp pinned beneath the ladder.

Thus, starting your third year is like going out into a blizzard with a windbreaker. Third year medical students are not only thrown into the clinical arena without an understanding of how to find out lab results, vitals or why you never under any circumstances page anyone but the intern; they are also thrown into direct patient contact. At that time, their interactions with patients can only be mediated by the discourse of the first two years of medical school, a discourse that really had little to do with patients. Hopefully, they had developed tools needed for sensitive interactions, or at least an appreciation of the importance of silence and thus the possibility of moments grounded in compassion. So the first day of the third year, students are to see their patients, typically not even knowing how to find the room numbers or a census list. Once they move beyond dealing with the practical details of medicine, they move onto the more nuanced realms of professional interaction, whether they recognize this or not.

On the wards, they will be subject to issues of professionalism from hazing by the nurses, impatience from all other members of the medical team and finally to eye rolling from everyone who is your senior . . . and everyone is. How to deal with this adjustment in the greater context of being a professional is never addressed in medical school. What then when faced with the overtired over-caffeinated senior resident or the even more fatigued and less experienced intern, the practical stressors, fatigue and a heavy patient load both practically and emotionally? Then discord prevails. Students at best have been given the theoretical context of professionalism without the intermediating discourse that fits their experience. They are left to fend for themselves or appeal to the nearest meaningful rubric handy. If grounded in a well articulated professional discourse, this is not troubling, but it rarely is. As most studies have shown, we appeal to that which surrounds us, identifying with our colleagues, and grasping the handiest context that will fit our situation, likely the disgruntled fourth-year student. What of compassion here? When we work to cultivate it in our patient interactions, it inevitably appears elsewhere, towards our colleagues, our senior staff and remarkably ourselves.

Unfortunately for students at this level of training, professionalism is positioned in the greater context of issues that rarely come up until they are at a much more senior level, and the opportunities to acquire the tools to work toward this goal are long gone. Professionalism in the clinical years is still in the realm of outside experts, experts who are unable to help students interpret the mundane details of daily experience. Even in a perfect system where students could articulate the values behind their commitment to professionalism in medicine, when those values are put to the test through real patient interaction, through late hours and the inordinate politics of any job, what then? Any ethical principles that were previously formed are meaningless without a meaningful commitment grounded in compassion to withstand the conflict and commentary that test them.

What to do

A means toward a solution can be seen in those programs that push students early to ground what is behind their commitment to medicine, and find language to articulate the gap between the theoretical and practical. For example, at the University of California–Irvine, pre-clinical medical students come up with their own codes of ethics, which allows them to come face to face, mediated through their own language, with the ways in which they expect to practice their profession (Cohn & Lie, 2002). The up side of this is that students have the opportunity to articulate their professional values. The down side of this is when, during their clinical education, those values are challenged not in an abstract manner but concretely via a real colleague or patient, students are no longer in contact with the group that helped make those values meaningful in the first place. Thus, students are left alone to determine these translations of the values into everyday practice, two years after their articulation.

Once medical education formally completes itself, and the lack of a bridge between the theoretical and practical realms of professional discourse has become a canyon, you move onto the formalized training of residency. There, training in professionalism goes little beyond the professed competency of an ACGME requirement. Those facilities that do train their residents in professionalism write articles about it and present this as research. That is, it is so remarkable, it is reportable. Strangely, at this level, professionalism has been returned not only to the sole domain of the medical professional, but even more specifically, it has been returned to the specialty area where the residency training takes place. Previously at the level of medical education, we deemed it important that other disciplines become involved in formation and development of professional values. But now that the formal portion of education has ended and the application of what has been learned is active, professionals are left to their own devices.

The limited literature in this area seems to indicate that tenets of professionalism do hold true: a true professional has an understanding of what needs to be done insofar it is done with technical acumen, and how it is to be done, that is, with a sensitivity to the greater personal, social and political context (Rowley et al., 2000). So good doctors will be good doctors, and isn't that where we started?

Although in this arena, the professional conflicts and ways in which we enact professionalism are somewhat different, the same problems still exist albeit on a different scale, since residents have more direct patient contact and impact than medical students. In short, things have come full circle: we have moved beyond theoretical formulations of what it is to be professional to the deeper commitments in practice that are required to sustain professionalism at this grueling level of training. I have attested throughout that without patient contact, professionalism is meaningless, and now in this unmediated realm of direct patient contact we have trusted, for better or worse, that professionals behave as they should. Even more surprising, we have found that our trust has been well placed.

In sum, the profession of medicine has fallen prey to other forces in articulating professionalism at a theoretical level. This has been made manifest in medical training. These forces have made positive contributions, particularly in the early years of medical training. Yet, medical trainees are progressively bereft of any professional guidance as they advance in their training and practice. This leaves them to adjudicate professionalism through the old lens of previous theoretical underpinnings and the new lens of the practice and the norms of those around them.

So we are standing over the patient, the machines are whirring and the chart is getting thicker and thicker with the notes and recommendations of consultants and results from lab tests that regardless of relevancy had to be ordered, but where is the patient? Amidst all of these interventions, the patient is not allowed to live or die. It is through this experience and this struggle that medical professionalism must come if it is to be meaningful rather than that afterthought of medical training.

In freeing itself from its interventions, I do not propose that we turn off all of the machines, turning our back of the progress of the theoretical contributions of professional theory. Instead, I think we should leave the ventilator on, keep the IVs running, but not merely for the sake of having them whir and drip. We need to look to the importance of professionalism as rooted in the recognition of what grounds the importance of medical practice. That is, there is something to medicine that does make the stakes just a little bit higher when we screw up, and this "something" needs to be communicated to medical students at all levels of training so they proceed to be good medical residents and practitioners. Of course I will argue that this "something" at stake is a consequence of the fact that another person is involved, a sick and vulnerable person. As a consequence of feeling and cultivating compassion for that person, we can recognize these higher stakes. With this initial recognition and assistance in articulating its formulation, professionalism is surely to follow.   Worse, as a failure of cultivating compassion, through its slow death, professionalism is just as likely to follow that fate.

REFERENCES

Beauchamp, T. C., & Childress, J. F. (1994). *Principles of biomedical ethics.* New York: Oxford University Press.
Cohn, F., & Lie, D. (2002). Mediating the gap between the white coat ceremony and the ethics and professionalism curriculum. *Academic Medicine, 77*(11), 1168.
Rowley, B. D., Baldwin, D. C., Jr., Bay, R. C., & Cannula, M. (2000). Can professional values be taught? A look at residency training. *Clinical Orthopaedics & Related Research, 378,* 110-114.
Starr, P. (1982). *The social transformation of American medicine.* New York: Basic Books.
Wear, D., & Castellani, B. (2000). The development of professionalism: Curriculum matters. *Academic Medicine, 75*(6), 602-611.

Chapter 12

WIT IS NOT ENOUGH

Audiey Kao and Jennifer Reenan
American Medical Association

WHY IS PROFESSIONALISM EDUCATION FAILING?

The Challenges of Low Demand and Unproven Supply

Western medicine was transformed by the intellectual revolution of eighteenth century Europe, also known as the Age of Enlightenment, which championed logic, reason, and the idea that the universe was orderly and ultimately comprehensible to the rational, observing mind. For thousands of years previously, medicine had been considered variously as a supernatural phenomenon, a spiritual practice and "a natural art" (Murray, 1998) whose practitioners were trained to assist nature with the healing process. Roy Porter (1997) describes pre-modern medicine in this way: "In the absence of decisive anatomical and physiological expertise and without a powerful arsenal of cures and surgical skills, the ability to diagnose and make prognoses was highly valued, and an intimate physician-patient relationship was fostered" (pp. 9-10). The novel "enlightened" philosophy of human inquiry subjected ancient conceptualizations of the body and disease, clinical intuition and instinct, and a variety of traditional therapeutic practices to the rigors and discipline of the scientific method. Ultimately, the Age of Enlightenment paved the way for the great scientific and technological discoveries and innovations of the last two centuries, which have led to dramatic advances in the diagnosis and treatment of diseases that have long afflicted humanity.

In the United States, the publication of the Flexner Report in 1910 further contributed to the rise and dominance of science in the practice of medicine and the training of its practitioners. This landmark report documented how many medical schools during that time failed to meet the basic requirements of an objective, science-based curriculum (Flexner, 1910). Informed by this data, state-licensing boards ultimately forced the closure of "doctor mills" that were producing inferior practitioners and sometimes, medical quacks. While this was a significant triumph in the history of medicine, the changes catalyzed by the Flexner Report led to the institutionalization of an educational system and medical culture that would be increasingly centered on the standardized application of the scientific method to the evaluation and treatment of diseases. Many advocates of scientific empiricism in medicine found that the "highest moral good was simply to master scientific medicine for the benefit of the patient" (Kenny, Mann, & MacLeod, 2003, p. 1205). The prototypic ideal physician of the post-Flexner era was poignantly portrayed by Sinclair Lewis in his 1925 novel *Arrowsmith*. Dr. Martin Arrowsmith, the novel's protagonist, works as a country doctor, a public health crusader and an inner-city hospitalist, but only becomes a truly heroic figure when he abandons his clinical work and adopts the ascetic, abstemious, and emotionally unattached life of a physician-scientist and researcher.

Despite the spectacular successes of science-based medicine in treating once fatal diseases, there is a widespread sense that the profession is in the midst of some sort of identity crisis. Bessinger (1988) notes that "there is a perception that medicine's science is at odds with medicine's art and with its sense of humanism" (p. 1558). Many contend that the benefits of the Flexnerian model of medical education and its focus on the hard sciences came at the expense of the "art" of medicine. As medicine became ever more closely aligned with the laws and methods of science, those aspects (e.g. psychological, cultural, social, and spiritual) of human illness and suffering which cannot be easily measured or submitted to scientific control and observation seemed less important or relevant to how we treat and interact with those who are sick and injured. The explosion of biomedical knowledge and technology has led to more hyper-specialization in clinical training and practice. As a result, it is often alleged that physicians view and treat their patients not as whole persons but as organ systems or disease states. Big science has also meant big business – forcing medicine to shed its humble roots as a caring and service-oriented vocation and become instead an occupation in which many view the patient-physician encounter as no different from any other economic transaction (Starr, 1982).

The profession has responded to this imbalance between the "art" and "science" of medicine by seeking to soften the edges of the Flexnerian model of medical education. In the early 1970s, courses and departments in medical ethics and the humanities began cropping up in U.S. medical schools (Hunter, Charon, & Coulehan, 1995; Miles, Weiss Lane, Bickel, Walker, & Cassel, 1989). Students needed exposure to these courses because biotechnology and commercial forces were dehumanizing medicine and giving rise to ethical dilemmas that science alone could not answer and that narrowly trained physicians were ill equipped to handle (Buxbaum, 1966; Pellegrino, 1974). Curricular changes designed to bolster the teaching of the art of medicine have fallen within various disciplines in the ensuing years and come under various course titles, including: ethics of medicine, introduction to doctoring, the art of physicianship, the doctor-patient relationship, medical humanities, medicine and society, and more recently (and most commonly in the present literature), professionalism.

Responding to the increasingly held public view that today's physicians are more technicians than healers, the goals of professionalism and other similar courses are to ensure that medical schools graduate compassionate and caring physicians. A typical professionalism course learning objective aims to cultivate "physician attitudes and actions that demonstrate interest in and respect for the patient and that address the patient's concerns and values" (Gracey et al., 2005, p. 22). Other intentions are to influence and shape physician attitudes and promote greater understanding of patients, colleagues, and self so as to stimulate more ethical decision making and professional behavior. Professionalism courses also stress the importance of teamwork, hoping to advance better intra- and inter-professional relationships in a health care learning and practice environment that for decades has been hypercompetitive and fragmented. Other commonly cited goals of professionalism curricula include increasing empathy and improving communication skills through an exploration of the ways that patients experience illness as depicted in literature, narratives, poetry, art, and theater. Understanding and developing strategies to cope with the complex social issues facing 21st century medicine, such as caring for the poor and uninsured, are yet other aims. All of these objectives reflect a general desire to "restore the heart and soul of medicine," which is widely viewed as being eroded by dehumanizing science and unchecked commercialism (Bonebakker, 2003). Yet, despite the growth in the number of professionalism courses in medical schools, concerns about the soul of the profession continue to be raised from both inside and outside medicine.

Why is professionalism education failing? Part of the answer to this question lies in the fact that there is low demand for these types of courses among medical students. This demand continues to drop throughout residency training and into clinical practice. Also, and probably more importantly, the supply of professionalism courses are of unproven educational value and effectiveness. Poorly designed and pedagogically flawed courses only serve to further dampen the demand and expectations of medical students for professionalism courses, creating a vicious cycle of low demand and unproven supply.

Given the institutionalization of science in medical education and training over the past century, it should not come as a surprise that the demand for professionalism courses among medical students is generally low. Many students consider professionalism courses to be unimportant or "touchy feely." It is also common to hear from students that these types of courses take time away from learning more relevant medical topics (American Medical Association, 2005). According to the AAMC's 2004 Graduation Questionnaire Summary Report, there is high demand among medical students for courses on subjects like practice management, pharmacogenetics and cost-effectiveness. Relatively few respondents indicated a need to devote more time to ethical decision-making and professionalism (AAMC, 2005). These views among medical students are most likely shared by some physician-educators who are not part of the "ethics" faculty, since their opinions are also shaped by their own personal experiences as medical students. Overall, the demand for professionalism instruction diminishes after medical school, as reflected by the fact that only a handful of states require continuing education on professionalism-related topics for medical licensure purposes.

In the marketplace of competing goods, the demand for a certain good is influenced by the perceived quality of that good. During the preclinical years of medical school, professionalism courses routinely involve large, didactic lectures taught by those who may have limited direct experience in the care of patients. When case-based learning is employed in these courses, the cases are typically designed to convey one specific topic (e.g. case on informed consent or privacy and confidentiality), and hence, lack many of the clinical and interpersonal details of a real world patient case. Other instructional methods such as role playing, poetry, fiction and patient narrative readings are also routinely used. But, how many William Carlos Williams poems does one have to read in order to learn how to communicate effectively with patients? Will attending a production of *Wit* really help a student be a more compassionate physician? While the goals of medical humanities and ethics courses are laudable, it is not clear that such learning activities have been successful in promoting the professionalism of future physicians. Given the views of many medical students that professionalism courses are less important or even irrelevant to good doctoring, professionalism courses of questionable effectiveness not only serve to amplify these negative perceptions among students, but also contribute to further reducing the demand. To be fair, questions about the educational quality of medical school curricula are certainly not limited to professionalism courses. There is a general lack of rigorous outcomes research to support the long term educational effectiveness of much of what is done in medical school (Carney et al., 2004). But basic science and clinical faculty do not have to deal with many of the supply side challenges faced by medical ethics and humanities faculty who often must justify the need for a better time slot and more resources for their curricular priorities.

If professionalism education is failing because of low demand and unproven supply, how can we start to address these challenges? We address this more fully in the remaining sections of this chapter. On the demand side, we start by defining professionalism in a manner that reaffirms the interdependent nature of the art and science of medicine. Given the tendency to compartmentalize the art and science of medicine within the curriculum, we believe that the way professionalism is currently defined and used only reinforces an unfortunate and "unnatural" division of the fundamental nature of the practice of medicine. It must be remembered that medicine in both the historical and living sense is not a science, as Murray (1998) points out, but rather "a caring profession that uses science." Indeed, medicine, at its core, is truly a humanistic (not scientific) endeavor as it seeks to defend and restore the integrity of the human body and human life. We would not pursue scientific and technological advances so fervently if we did not value human life and our common humanity so passionately.

Medical students and physicians must appreciate or remember that to be a good doctor requires not only scientific knowledge and technical skills, but also ethical awareness and psychosocial understanding. Just as physicians apply modern science to help their patients, medical ethics and humanities education provide tools and strategies that can be applied, in a practical sense, to the practice of good medicine. Students who are regularly exposed to a splintered conceptualization of medicine will fail to grasp fully what it means to be a physician in service to people who are sick and vulnerable. With greater appreciation of professionalism, students will demand more of their educational career, and in turn, teachers of medicine will be challenged and inspired to respond with improved course offerings in a positive learning environment.

To address the supply side challenges, we must first identify the limitations and weaknesses of current professionalism curricula as it has been narrowly defined by many educators. Recognizing that every medical school is slightly different, it is important that we reach consensus on some basic "design principles" that are critical to the development and implementation of educationally effective curricula and that are in keeping with a broader definition of professionalism, which we present in the next section of the chapter. In the final section of this chapter, we will examine eight key curricular design principles for improving instructional and assessment methods in professionalism education.

WHAT IS PROFESSIONALISM IN MEDICINE?

Reaffirming the Interdependence of the Art and Science in Good Doctoring

Professional, n.: one who has an assured competence in a particular field or occupation.

-ism, suffix: (1) A characteristic behavior or quality for example, heroism or individualism. (2) An action, practice, or process; for example, terrorism or favoritism. (3) A doctrine, theory, system, or principle; for example, capitalism or expressionism. (American Heritage Dictionary, 1976, pp. 694, 1045)

When we speak of professionalism in medicine, it is fair to say that we are not all talking about the same concept. As we noted earlier, professionalism has been increasingly used as another way of referring to the art or ethics of medicine. This narrower characterization of professionalism is probably most notably conveyed by the Accreditation Council for Graduate Medical Education (ACGME), which sets and enforces standards for residency training programs in medicine. According to the ACGME, professionalism is one of six competencies in which physician trainees in accredited residency programs must demonstrate assured competence (ACGME, 2001). However, there are others who view professionalism in medicine through a more robust competence lens. According to Epstein and Hundert (2002), professional competence in medicine is the "habitual and judicious use of communication, knowledge, technical skills, clinical reasoning, emotions, values, and reflection in daily practice for the benefit of the individual and community being served" (p. 226). We favor this broader, semantically more accurate definition of professionalism. Professionalism in medicine is, then, *the maintenance of competencies essential to the practice, teaching, and advancement of science-based, ethical, and compassionate care in service to patients and society.*

From a clinical perspective, a definition of professionalism in medicine that is based on the acquisition and maintenance of competencies essential for sustaining the art and science of care may prompt the criticism that such a broad conceptualization tries to capture everything that is important in good doctoring. We agree and, in fact, see this potential "critique" as strength. It is our contention that medical education is fundamentally professionalism education. From the first days of medical school (and many believe even before then), medical students embark on a process of professionalization that socializes them to be lifelong learners who strive to maintain continuing professional competence in all of those areas required for the delivery of high quality care to patients and society. Given the emphasis that we place on the science of medicine, it is sobering to realize that much of the clinical information and technical skills that students learn during their undergraduate career will be outdated at some point during their clinical practice. Therefore, professionalism education, especially during the formative years of a physician's educational career, must focus less on memorizing facts, and more on providing learners with knowledge (e.g. medical informatics, health economics, and epidemiology) and skills, while striving to hardwire professional attitudes (e.g. continual pursuit of clinical excellence) and conduct that prepare physicians to deliver quality care throughout their professional life. It is worth noting that while our broader conceptualization of professionalism, like other definitions, deals with physicians in their role as clinician, it is also more comprehensive, recognizing the other "hats" that physicians wear as teacher and mentor, scientist and researcher, and citizen and advocate.

At this point, many readers may be wondering why we have placed so much emphasis on the semantics and definition of professionalism. It may seem like a pedantic exercise, especially if most educators already agree upon and use professionalism in a narrowly construed fashion. We respectfully disagree that accurately defining professionalism, even in the context of majority dissent, is a trivial pursuit. Human ideas are conveyed through words, and as such, how we define and use words and language is essential to any successful endeavor. We fully appreciate that others, including possibly chapter authors in this book, may refer to professionalism in a manner put forth by the ACGME. We urge serious reconsideration of how, as educators, we define and conceptualize professionalism. As we noted earlier, the use of a definition of professionalism that does not acknowledge the full range of necessary competencies only serves to aggravate the curricular compartmentalization of the art and science of medicine, and contribute to the marginalization of instruction in ethical knowledge and interpersonal skills that are important for good doctoring. A broader conceptualization of professionalism is not only semantically more accurate than the narrower definition accepted by many medical educators, but it is also instrumentally and normatively more valid and compelling.

From an instrumental perspective, medical professionalism requires that a physician possess scientific knowledge and technical expertise as well as the ethical and interpersonal skills needed to deliver high quality medical care. Given medicine's increasing ability to treat diseases and keep people alive, a physician must know not only how to diagnose accurately and treat effectively, but also how to communicate well with patients, work toward understanding their values and preferences, and, in this age of high-tech medicine, when to stop treating and focus on palliation and comfort. In practice, the art and science of medicine are interdependent in that, for example, one's ability to provide technically competent care in part is dependent on one's ability to communicate with patients.

Let's say you are presented with a choice of a surgeon who has stellar technical skills, but communicates poorly with patients, and another who has average technical skills, but possesses excellent bedside manners. Who would you choose? This hypothetical scenario presents a false choice because there is no reason why a patient should have to settle for a technically superior surgeon who has poor communication skills and bedside manner. Even a surgeon who has extraordinary technical skills can make a mistake and, in these circumstances, will have to rely on the ability to communicate with patients and families and, maybe more importantly, will have to draw on the good interpersonal relationship that was established prior to the medical error. Studies have shown that patients' satisfaction with their medical care is dependent on more than just the technical aspects of their clinical experience (Little et al., 2001). From an instrumental perspective, therefore, the ability to deliver good medical care is grounded in the interdependent nature of the art and science of medicine.

That the art and science of medicine are interdependent does not presuppose a specific proportionality of importance between the two in the provision of good medical care. Prior to modern scientific advances in medicine, the artful practice of medicine was the primary therapy a physician had to offer a sick or dying patient. Since the arrival of such advances as antibiotics, diagnostic radiology, trauma care, and organ transplantation, the "pendulum" has swung toward a more scientific approach to disease and more limited view of patients and their suffering (Charon, 2000). Only a fool would wish to return to a time when medicine was practiced without the advantages of modern science. A definition of medical professionalism that does not acknowledge the pre-eminence of science will ring hollow to medical students and practicing physicians. Scientific knowledge and technical competence are of great consequence to both physicians and patients and, for many if not most, of the greatest consequence. But the highest moral good of medicine is not the mastery of scientific and technical knowledge, even if it is to the benefit of fellow human beings. The practice of medicine means more than just applying science to disease. Physicians are pivotal characters in the life stories of many and if, in our zest for science, we mistakenly believe that it provides us with all of the answers to the human condition, we have failed our patients. The challenge for medical educators is to incorporate a curriculum that recognizes the interdependence of art and science for the practice of good medicine.

From a sociological perspective, professions are defined communities of individuals that are bound by and share common features and characteristics. First, a profession like medicine has a defined set of knowledge and skills. Second, a true profession has an established code of ethical conduct. Third, a profession strives to uphold the integrity of self-regulation because it is argued that those in the profession can best determine whether individual members have deviated from accepted standards of competence and conduct. According to Cruess, Johnston, and Cruess (2004), a profession is an occupation whose core elements is work based upon the mastery of a complex body of knowledge and skills. It is a vocation in which knowledge of some department of science or learning or the practice of an art founded upon it is used in the service of others. Its members are governed by codes of ethics; they profess a commitment to competence, integrity and morality, altruism, and the promotion of the public good within their domain. These commitments form the basis of a social contract between a profession and society, which in return grants the profession a monopoly over the use of its knowledge base, the right to considerable autonomy in practice and the privilege of self-regulation. Professions and their members are accountable to those served and to society (Cruess, Johnston, & Cruess, 2004, p. 75).

This understanding of profession draws from the extensive literature from scholars and theorists exploring the sociology of professions (Friedson, 1994; Larson, 1977; Parsons, 1939; Wilensky, 1964). It is important to note that, according to this body of work, all professions, including medicine, are expected to define a body of competence for members of the profession, and must ensure that practitioners are proficient. This body of competence is not limited to technical skills, but also includes the proviso that "practice of an art founded upon it is used in the service of others" (Cruess, Johnston, & Cruess, 2004, p. 75). Hence, our definition of professionalism in medicine is properly derived from this sociological interpretation of the meaning of profession.

THE WHO, WHEN, WHERE, AND HOW OF PROFESSIONALISM EDUCATION: DESIGN PRINCIPLES FOR NURTURING THE LEARNING ENVIRONMENT IN MEDICINE

Taking a journalistic approach, we have asked and attempted to answer "why" and "what" questions concerning the state of professionalism education in the first half of this chapter. In this final section, we examine the "who, when, where, and how" questions with the goal of outlining key curriculum design principles that must be incorporated in establishing a learning environment that supports professionalism education during the medical school years and beyond.

Who Should Teach Professionalism? See One, Do One, Teach One

Design principle #1: Teachers of medical students should only include those who have the demonstrated ability to present, frame, and reinforce those competencies essential to the practice of science-based, ethical, and compassionate care.

If the primary goal of professionalism education is to produce physicians that can provide the best possible care, who should be responsible for preparing and training these future physicians for clinical excellence? The answer seems straightforward and simple enough: It should be individuals who have experience and expertise in providing high quality care to patients. Put another way, it is difficult if not impossible, for a teacher to impart a technical skill to a novice or for a novice to learn reasoned judgment from a teacher, if the teacher has never seen, performed or practiced it herself. Therefore, medical schools require capable physician-educators who have demonstrated achievement in their respective specialties and can be effective teachers and role models of good doctoring and medical professionalism.

For much of history, it was believed that medical students could learn how to be good doctors largely by observing and helping experienced doctors practice medicine. Even after the establishment of medical schools, the apprenticeship model of learning continued to be an important conduit for transmitting professional values and skills. This tradition of role modeling as a means of imparting professionalism relied heavily on the ancient notion of virtue. Rooted in the philosophical writings of Plato and Aristotle, virtue ethics centers on the importance of one's innate moral character (or the type of person one is) and, in the practical sense, implies that virtues such as compassion and altruism can be cultivated through the habitual "doing" of good deeds (Gardiner, 2003). Such habits are informed by observing and mimicking more experienced physicians, a practice now commonly referred to as "shadowing" or "situated learning" (Lave & Wegner, 1991). In their recent and influential work on the "hidden curriculum," Hafferty and Franks (1994) describe the powerful impact that more senior physicians, even outside the classroom and formal learning environment, have on the professional development of medical students and resident physicians.

If we accept the premise that experienced physicians should be the primary teachers of medical students, then what is the role, if any, of the research biochemist or the moral philosopher in medical professionalism education? What does a teacher with a Ph.D. in biochemistry or literature know about being a physician, about taking care of sick patients at the end of life, or breaking bad news to family members? Can they realistically be expected to present, convey, and reinforce medical professionalism, integrating both the art and science, to students and resident physicians? Some may say that it would be better to have physicians who have additional, specialized training outside the field of medicine teach non-clinical subjects like biochemistry, ethics, or statistics. If the main goal of medicine is ultimately to serve patients, it seems as though students would benefit most from those who know what it is like to care for patients and who can appropriately apply the liberal arts and the basic sciences into fulfilling the primary goals of medicine.

While this physician-only stance may have some appeal, non-physician scientists and ethicists have valuable knowledge and insights to impart to medical students. Yet medical school faculty who ask students to memorize the steps of the Krebs cycle are not advancing the goals of professionalism education in medicine, just as having a philosopher serve as the course director for the major (and possibly only) ethics course in medical school can send the wrong signal to medical students about the importance of the content. Most physicians are not scientists and would not consider themselves as such, nor are they academic humanists. Teachers of medicine, physician or not, who are pedagogically inflexible and myopic will make it extremely difficult to realize the primary goals of medical or professionalism education. The bottom line for all faculty is to impart information and insights in a manner that is instrumental to good doctoring and appropriate to the developmental stage of the learner.

When Should Professionalism Be Taught?

Design principle #2: Given that professional attitudes and conduct of future physicians are shaped early in their educational careers, curricula designed to promote the art of medicine must be implemented throughout medical school with particular emphasis on the clinical years.

While our conceptualization of professionalism affirms the interdependent nature of the art and science of medicine, we must still ask when during medical school years should these two content pillars be emphasized. Why is the "when" question important to address? First, as we noted earlier, much of the scientific truths and technical skills that one learns in medical school will be found to be wrong or outdated during one's professional career. Second, we know from the literature on moral development that the early years of professionalism education greatly shape the lifelong potential of physicians to deliver ethical and compassionate patient care (Crain, 1985). Taken together, these two basic assumptions force one to ask, when in a physician's education should the ethics and compassion of professional competency be introduced and when should the science-based knowledge that is also essential to professional competency be emphasized?

Wear and Kuczewski (2004) have pointed out that many "students enter medical school already full of the values espoused by the profession" (p. 6). In fact, the majority of premedical students receive significant exposure to the humanities during their college years, and a significant percentage of accepted medical school applicants majored in a liberal arts discipline (Niemi & Phillips, 1980). Despite that, many medical students are less humanistic and more cynical when they graduate then when they entered school (Coulehan & Williams, 2001). Given that the formation of one's professional attitudes and conduct occurs in such an early and narrow time frame, professionalism curricula that emphasize the art of medicine should be front-loaded with special emphasis during the clinical years of medical school and residency training. It is more difficult, and some would say impossible, to expect to alter a physician's attitudes and conduct at the back end after he or she has been in practice for many years.

Currently, most ethics courses are taught in the pre-clinical years of medical school, with relatively little formal attention to these matters during the required clinical clerkships and elective rotations when the potential negative impact of the hidden curriculum on professional attitudes and conduct are probably highest. The current trend to expose first and second year medical students to the clinics, the hospital wards, and private medical practice, only underscores the fact that attention to and emphasis on instilling the art of medicine in the earliest years of a physician's lifelong learning career are critical. With that said, we are not implying that basic science education in the first two years should be eliminated, but rather it needs to better designed and integrated with the other dimensions of professionalism, such as through more problem-based learning. Nevertheless, there may be only a brief window of opportunity to influence positively and lastingly a physician's professional attitudes and conduct. In contrast, expectations for competency in and knowledge of the biomedical sciences will be constantly changing and evolving. It has been estimated that to keep up with new knowledge and maintain currency in their own specialty, the average physician would need to read at least seventeen articles per day (Davidoff, Haynes, Sackett, & Smith, 1995). There is simply no educational rationale for "cramming in" scientific information during the early years of medical training that will likely have little, if any, direct relevance and value to the current or future practice of medicine.

Where Should Professionalism Be Taught?

Design principle #3: Teachers of medicine must recognize that learning occurs outside the traditional settings, and that therefore, they should develop ways of expanding their educational reach into these other venues.

For medical students, professionalism education occurs in settings that go well beyond the lecture hall, laboratory bench, or conference room. Whether it is in the hallways after rounds, in the anatomy lab locker room, at lunch in the hospital cafeteria, or sometimes even in social settings such as the local breakfast joint or neighborhood bar, professional attitudes and conduct are being shaped and learned. Hundert (1996) refers to the many professionally formative experiences that occur well outside of formal classroom settings, which he refers to as the informal curriculum. Indeed, he reports that "the vast majority of the situations the students described as the most influential were conversations with no faculty present. These often happened over lunch or dinner or just *after* a course" (p. 625). If professionalism education is happening in almost every place where students are interacting with other students, educators must expand the "walls" of their classroom to encompass this complex learning environment.

It is important that we develop ways to engage the learner in these non-traditional settings where learning is occurring because, otherwise, the educational objectives of the formal curriculum will be undermined. This will not be easy to accomplish given that it is impossible for teachers of medicine to be everywhere medical students work, live, and play. One small but tangible example, that most of us are familiar with, involves the signs that are placed in the public spaces of an academic health center (e.g. elevators and cafeteria) that stress the importance of not openly discussing the medical details of patient cases or making personal comments about patients themselves. Another growing trend is the establishment of virtual classrooms that create a new space where medical students can reflect and converse with their peers and their teachers (see, for example, Inui et al. in this book). Of course, more research and attention must be directed to assess the educational value of these virtual classrooms and similar efforts to expand the reach of professionalism education beyond the physical classroom. Therefore, the question that teachers of medicine must address becomes less "where should professionalism be taught," but "how they can strive to be in the non-traditional places where professionalism is being learned?"

How Should Professionalism be Taught and Evaluated?

We now turn our attention to what is probably the most challenging question in medical professionalism education: how should it be taught and evaluated? In a culture of academic health centers, where the educational mission often seems overshadowed by the drive for increased revenue and prestige from patient care and biomedical research, teachers of medicine do not have the luxury of being inefficient and ineffective in their efforts to educate and train the next generation of physicians. With persistent, inappropriate variations in clinical decision making and declining trust in physicians and the profession, it is fair to say that we have yet to realize an educational system that eliminates the physician-dependent factor among the multi-factorial causes of medical disparities and mistrust. As has been noted already, there is little evidence that professionalism education has been successful in producing more ethical and compassionate physicians (Shapiro, Morrison, & Boker, 2004). Medical education leaders are keenly aware of this reality. Indeed, Branch et al. (2001) argue that "many currently used strategies to induce humanism are probably ineffective" (p. 1073); other observers note that "the literature advocating for use of the arts as a desirable teaching method remains largely anecdotal and unsystematic" (Rodenhauser, Strickland, & Gambala, 2004, p. 237). Curricular changes and reforms that have little outcomes evidence to support their continuing utilization and widespread adoption have contributed to "a history of reform without change, of repeated modifications of the medical school curriculum that alter very slightly, or not at all, the experience of the critical participants, the students and teachers" (Bloom, 1998, p. 295). From this chaotic environment, we offer some final design principles that along with those presented earlier will hopefully serve as a compass for guiding quality professionalism education.

Design principle #4: Professionalism competencies are categorized into knowledge, skills, judgment, and behaviors, and each medical specialty has to reach consensus on how these competency categories manifest in the practice of science-based, ethical, and compassionate care in their specialty.

From an instructional and assessment perspective, we consider professionalism competencies to be those aspects of good doctoring, including both the art and science of medicine, that are teachable and learnable, but are also testable and assessable. For example, an internist must possess specific clinical (e.g. causes of ketoacidosis) and ethical (e.g. components of proper informed consent) knowledge; a general surgeon must demonstrate certain technical (e.g. surgical suturing ability) and communication skills (e.g. how to deliver bad news to families); a pediatrician must be able to come to the right decision, based on reasoned judgment (e.g. determine whether or not to report a parent to child protective services); and a psychiatrist must learn to behave professionally with patients (e.g. act in a manner to maintain proper boundaries between the patient and the physician). Within each specialty, consensus must be reached on how these competency categories manifest in the practice of science-based, ethical, and compassionate care in their specialty. However, this is not to suggest that professionalism competencies are all specialty specific. Of course, there are competencies that apply to all physicians regardless of specialty (e.g. communication skills and proper conduct with patients, peers, and colleagues), and this must be part of the curriculum for all medical students. There must be collective agreement within the profession in general as well as within specialties about what professionalism is and what it encompasses before we can develop truly effective professionalism curricula.

Not only do professionalism competencies have to be teachable and learnable, they also must be testable and assessable. For example, medical knowledge is typically evaluated in a written examination; skills such as communications can be assessed by utilizing standardized patients (Barrows, 1993); judgment is typically evaluated retrospectively during morning rounds and in morbidity and mortality conferences; and conduct is usually observable by teachers of medicine in various setting such as the wards and classrooms. Currently, available assessment methods remain largely subjective and invalidated, and therefore, more medical education research needs to be conducted in this critical area (Arnold, 2002; Epstein & Hundert, 2002).

Design principle #5: Given the interdependent nature of the art and science of medicine, formal and informal means of instruction in professionalism competencies must strive to integrate these two pillars of good doctoring in its pedagogy.

As we have already noted earlier in this chapter, the practice of good medicine requires scientific knowledge and technical skills, as well as ethical awareness and psychosocial abilities. One of the problems of having compartmentalized courses on the art and the science of medicine is the marginalization of the former, to the detriment of the latter given the interdependent nature of the two. However, promising methods of formal instruction, like standardized patient exercises (Barrows, 1993) and problem-based learning (Roche, Scheetz, Dane, Parish, & O'Shea, 2003), have the potential to present the competencies relevant to both the art and science of medicine in a more integrated manner. Instruction using standardized patients provides a unique opportunity to train medical students in a tangible way about the interdependent nature of the art and science of medicine. Problem-based learning was developed, in many ways, to deal with the over-compartmentalized, discipline-oriented instruction that was the norm for the preclinical years of medical school up until the early 1990's. Recently, problem-based learning has also served as an educational platform for the integration of various professionalism competencies.

Efforts to integrate the instructional content on the informal side presents its own unique challenges in that it depends, in many ways, on the everyday actions and mentoring abilities of clinical faculty, some of who may not fully appreciate the interdependent nature of the art and science of medicine. Many medical schools have established "academies" that recognize the best teachers, and some have also begun to initiate more faculty development programs that aim to train attending physicians to be better teachers, mentors, and role models (Jones & Verghese, 2003; Shapiro & Rucker, 2003). Unfortunately, these types of initiatives are usually under-funded in medical schools and residency programs, and therefore, greater efforts should be made to capitalize and nurture these new and emerging educational innovations.

Design principle #6: Instruction in professionalism competencies must be contextually relevant and appropriate to the educational stage of the learner.

As adult learners, medical students share many of the same characteristics as those aspiring to achieve competency in other fields and occupations. These characteristics include: 1) a tendency towards independent, autonomous and self-directed learning, 2) a need to connect their practical, life experiences with learned theories and concepts, 3) a need to set and achieve concrete goals, and 4) a desire for learning that is *relevant*, practical and useful to their work or area of interest (Lieb, 2005). According to Knowles (1976), who identified these key characteristics, adult learners use their own personal and professional experiences to establish educational goals; this idea should inform consideration of how medical students might respond to professionalism education.

Relevancy is extremely important to medical students because they are confronted with competing time demands. As such, it is critical that learning activities be considered of value or they will be ignored, brushed through or hastily forgotten. Thus, learning activities that are context-based and interactive are more likely to affect physician behavior as well as patient outcomes (Davis et al., 1999). As Eggly, Brennan and Wiese-Rometsch (2005) argue in their recent article aptly titled "Once when I was on call...: Theory versus Reality in Training for Professionalism," the "challenge to physicians and medical educators is to set standards, teach and assess professional behavior in a way that converges with and builds upon trainees' daily experiences" (p. 372). Analyzing the writings of interns at a large academic health center, these authors found that medical trainees have a strong preoccupation with the interpersonal aspects of their work, especially the physician-patient relationship. To make professionalism topics relevant to this cohort, it may be necessary to link abstract principles to real-life experiences with patients.

The importance of relevancy requires medical educators to examine critically many existing learning activities in medical professionalism. Professionalism education must focus on teaching those competencies that ensure that medical students can practice science-based, ethical, and compassionate medicine throughout their professional life. Teachers must be prepared to explain and defend professionalism education activities in terms of the everyday work that physicians do. Frankly, it is doubtful that elective courses like "Medicine and Victorian Culture" or "Sherlock Holmes and Clinical Judgment" will appeal to the majority of medical students in a given class. Expending finite resources on well-intentioned educational activities that fail the relevancy test is costly, both financially and instructionally.

Design principle #7: Professionalism education must provide medical students with opportunities for personal reflection and self-directed learning in order for them to become successful lifelong learners.

While we have focused on professionalism education in medical school, these four years of schooling represents the beginning, and not the end of a physician's learning career. Professionalism is the acquisition and *maintenance* of competencies essential for good doctoring, and that requires continual learning and re-learning. Reflective practices and self-directed learning can develop the capacities and hardwire the habits that are critical for good doctoring and professional satisfaction (Frankford, Patterson, & Konrad, 2000;Epstein, 1999). However, the medical education system has not spent much effort in creating the time, space, and conditions necessary for learners to effectively process and openly discuss their experiences with peers and teachers.

As the profession works towards reaching consensus on what the professionalism competencies are and how they should be imparted in medical education, the perspectives of students should be seriously considered by teachers of medicine. A central feature of self-directed learning is that the learner must assume some responsibility for setting and realizing the learning goals. From an educational perspective, creating opportunities for medical students to reflect on their experiences and learn from them such as through keeping a journal, participating in safe, small group conversation (Branch, 2001), and organizing student interest groups can create opportunities for learning and growth in many aspects of professionalism. These activities may require fewer resources than many existing medical school courses and can offer the added benefit of helping medical students cope with stress, shed light on inappropriate norms in the learning environment, and serve as an important signal to medical students that their voice matters.

Design principle #8: Assessment of professionalism competencies must be timely, valid, and be provided from multiple perspectives. Such assessment must include long term evaluation of medical students' ability to practice science-based, ethical, and compassionate care.

Compared to instructional efforts, methods of assessing professionalism competencies lag well behind in their development and progress. Many reasons have contributed to this assessment gap including lack of clarity and consensus on the set of competencies that should be measured, a perception that one cannot measure certain aspects of professionalism in an objective and quantitative manner, and, until recently, lower expectations from accreditation bodies of medical schools and residency programs to more fully address competency attainment by students and resident physicians. But since the establishment of ACGME's "core competency" requirements and maintenance of certification efforts by various specialty boards, there has been growing attention on how better to assess the continuing professional competency of physicians.

First, assessment of professionalism competencies needs to be timely in order to provide the learner with the opportunity to respond constructively to critical feedback. However, there is some feedback that is more "time-sensitive" from a continuum of learning perspective. As we noted earlier, much of the science of medicine that students acquire will become irrelevant at some point in their practice. Assessment of scientific knowledge, technical skills and clinical judgment, therefore, is a critical enterprise that extends well beyond the medical school years. However, professionalism competencies such as communication skills and ethical conduct are generally acquired during a relatively short and early time period in a physician's professional life, and thus, it is necessary that medical educators determine whether a student has acquired these competencies.

Medical educators have yet to determine how best to assess the humanistic aspects of professionalism. Misch (2002) asks whether "humanism [should] be assessed solely on the basis of behavior, or must a physician's knowledge . . . [in this domain] be measured so as to provide a full and valid evaluation?"(p. 490). While this question is an important methodological question, it is probably fair to say that there is no method that can fully assess whether one has acquired the essential competencies of good doctoring. In the absence of a "one size fits all" measure, many assessment methods are being used or have been proposed, including individual direct observation by faculty or residents, standardized patient evaluations, self-assessment forms, "humanism connoisseurs" (Misch, 2002, p. 491), quantitative rating scales, qualitative commentary, and peer evaluation forms.

Medical education research on the validity of different assessment methods needs to be conducted. One important research area is determining who the best judge of different aspects of professionalism competencies is. Not so long ago, the only individuals providing assessment of medical student performance were senior, more experienced physicians. While this will undoubtedly remain the single, most important evaluation source, others including nurses and other allied health professionals, peers, and patients, real or simulated, may provide more relevant and valid assessment for specific professionalism competencies such as communication skills. For example, the use of standardized patients to evaluate how well a student can deliver bad news is increasingly being employed in medical schools. The adoption of innovative assessment methods such as standardized patients is a far cry from the days when medical students were simply sent into a hospital to conduct medical interview, with very little feedback and critique from patients on the quality of the encounter. More research on the value of multiple assessors will inform educators on how better to develop and implement assessment systems in medical schools.

CONCLUSIONS: BEYOND MEDICAL SCHOOL

Beyond the challenges of professionalism education in medical school, ensuring the maintenance of competencies during a physician's professional life presents even greater hurdles. Medical students are "captive" learners, and teachers regularly engage them in formal learning environments, but there are no traditional classrooms for practicing physicians, and there is no teacher who is watching over them. Questions about what should be the core elements of a lifelong curriculum for physicians are not fully answered. Who should and how to effectively assess that physicians continually possess the competencies to deliver quality patient care remain largely unresolved. Addressing these and other challenges is critical because physicians are students of medicine for life, but only medical students for a relatively brief period in their professional career.

Like all professions, medicine has long possessed special rights and privileges that are recognized by society. This cherished status is grounded in the expectation that professions will ensure that its practitioners are competent in carrying out its craft. As we approach the 100th anniversary of the Flexner report, the medical profession recognizes that the time has arrived to fundamentally examine how physicians acquire and maintain the knowledge, skills, behavior, and judgment essential to the delivery of ethical, science-based, and compassionate care, and to make the necessary changes to strengthen the three stages of the educational *continuum*— medical school, residency training and fellowship, and continuing physician professional development. A concerted effort to change the culture of medicine and transform the infrastructure to support and promote lifelong learning and constructive assessment must be undertaken, lest parties outside of medicine deem it appropriate for them to intervene. With such a profession-wide commitment to promote excellence in patient care through advances in physician learning, the medical profession will reaffirm its obligation to advocate for the sick and injured, and, in turn, strengthens the public's trust in medicine.

The views expressed in this chapter are those of the authors and are not necessarily those of their affiliated organization.

REFERENCES

Accreditation Council for Graduate Medical Education (ACGME). (2001). *Outcomes project.* Retrieved July 8, 2005 from ACGME website: http://www.acgme.org

American Medical Association Step Program. (2005). Unpublished qualitative data.

Association of American Medical Colleges (AAMC). (2005). Medical school graduation questionnaire, 1978-2005. Retrieved July 27, 2005 from AAMC website: http://www.aamc.org/data/gq/

Arnold, L. (2002). Assessing professional behavior: Yesterday, today, and tomorrow. *Academic Medicine, 77,* 502-515.

Barrows, H.S. (1993). An overview of the uses of standardized patients for teaching and evaluating clinical skills. *Academic Medicine, 68,* 443-451.

Bessinger, C.D. (1988). Doctoring: The philosophic milieu. *Southern Medical Journal, 81,* 1558-1562.

Bloom, S.W. (1998). Structure and ideology in medical education: An analysis of resistance to change. *Journal of Health and Social Behavior, 29,* 294-306.

Bonebakker, V. (2003). Literature and medicine: Humanities at the heart of health care. *Academic Medicine, 78,* 963-967.

Branch, W.T. (2001). Small group teaching emphasizing reflection can positively influence medical students' values. *Academic Medicine, 76,* 1171-1172.

Branch, W.T., Kern, D., Haidet, P., Weissman, P., Gracey, C.F., Mitchell, G., et al. (2001). Teaching the human dimensions of care in clinical settings. *Journal of the American Medical Association, 286,* 1067-1074.

Buxbaum, R.C. (1966). Toward human values in medical practice. *Journal of Medical Education, 41*, 516-520.

Carney, P.A., Nierenberg, D.W., Pipas, C.F., Brooks, W.B., Stukel, T.A., Keller, A.M. (2004). Educational epidemiology: Applying population-based design and analytic approaches to study medical education. *Journal of the American Medical Association, 292*, 1044-1050.

Charon, R. (2000). Literature and medicine: Origins and destinies. *Academic Medicine, 75*, 23-27.

Coulehan, J., & William, P.C. (2001). Vanquishing virtue: The impact of medical education. *Academic Medicine, 76*, 5998-605.

Crain, W.C. (1985). *Theories of development*. Englewood Cliffs, NJ: Prentice-Hall.

Cruess, S.R., Johnston, S., & Cruess, R.L. (2004). Profession: A working definition for medical educators. *Teaching and Learning in Medicine, 16*, 74-76.

Davidoff, R., Haynes, R.B., Sackett, D.L., & Smith, R. (1995). Evidence based medicine: A new journal to help doctors identify the information that they need. *BMJ, 310*, 1085-1086.

Davis, E., O'Brien, M.A., Freemantle, N., Wolf, F.M., Mazmanian, P., & Taylor-Vaisey, A. (1999). Impact of formal continuing medical education: Do conferences, workshops, rounds, and other traditional continuing educational activities change physician behavior or health outcomes? *Journal of the American Medical Association, 282*, 867-874.

Eggly, S., Brenna, S., & Wiese-Rometsch, W. (2005). "Once when I was on call . . . .": Theory versus reality in training for professionalism. *Academic Medicine, 80*, 371-375.

Epstein, R.M. (1999). Mindful practice. *The Journal of the American Medical Association, 282*(9), 833-839.

Epstein, R.M., & Hundert, E.M. (2002). Defining and assessing professional competence. *JAMA, 287*, 226-235.

Flexner, A. (1910). *Medical education in the United States and Canada*. New York: Carnegie Foundation for the Advancement of Teaching.

Frankford, D.M., Patterson, M.A., & Konrad, T.R. (2000). Transforming the practice organizations to foster lifelong learning and commitment to medical professionalism. *Acadaemic Medicine, 2000*, 708-717.

Friedson, E. (1994). *Professionalism reborn*. Chicago: University of Chicago Press.

Gardiner, P. (2003). A virtue ethics approach to moral dilemmas in medicine. *Journal of Medical Ethics, 29*, 297-302.

Gracey, C.F., Haidet, P., Branch, W.T., Weissmann, P., Kern, D.E., Mitchell, G., et al. (2005). Precepting humanism: Strategies for fostering the human dimensions of care in ambulatory settings. *Academic Medicine, 80*, 21-28.

Hafferty, F., & Franks, R. (1991) The hidden curriculum, ethics teaching and the structure of medical education. *Academic Medicine, 69*, 861-871.

Hundert, E.M. (1996). Characteristics of the informal curriculum and trainees' ethical choices. *Academic Medicine, 71*, 624-633.

Hunter, K.M., Charon, R., & Coulehan, J.L. (1995). The study of literature in medical education. *Academic Medicine, 70*, 787-794.

Jones, T., & Verghese, A. (2003). On becoming a humanities curriculum: The Center for Medical Humanities and Ethics at the University of Texas Health Science Center at San Antonio. *Academic Medicine, 78*, 1010-1014.

Kenny, N.P., Mann, K.V., & MacLeod, H. (2003). Role modeling in physicians' professional formation: Reconsidering an essential but untapped educational strategy. *Academic Medicine, 78*, 1203-1210.

Knowles, M. (1996). Andradgogy: An emerging technology for adult learning. In R. Edwards, A. Hanson, & P. Raggatt (Eds.), *Boundaries of adult learning* (pp. 82-98). New York: Routledge.

Larson, M. (1977). *The rise of professionalism: A sociological analysis.* Berkeley: University of California Press.

Lave, J., & Wegner, E. (1991). *Situated learning: Legitmate peripheral participation.* Cambridge: Cambridge University Press.

Lewis, S. (1925). *Arrowsmith.* New York: Harcourt, Brace.

Lieb, S. (2001). Principles of adult learning. Retrieved April 15, 2005 from the University of Hawaii website: http://www.hcc.hawaii.edu/intranet/committees/FacDevCom/guidebk/teachtip/adults-2.htm

Little, P., Everitt, H., Williamson, I., Warner, G., Moore, M., Gould, C., et al. (2001). Preferences of patients for patient centered approach to consultation in primary Care: Observational study. *BMJ, 322*, 468-472.

Miles, S., Weiss Lane, L. Bickel, J., Walker, R., & Cassel, C. (1989). Medical ethics education: Coming of age. *Academic Medicine, 64*, 705-714.

Misch, D.A. (2002). Evaluating physicians' professionalism and humanism: The case for humanism "connoisseurs." *Academic Medicine, 77*, 489-495.

Murray, T.J. (1998, June). Why the medical humanities? *The Dalhousie Medical Journal.* Retrieved April 26, 2005 from the website: http://medjournal.medicine.dal.ca/DMJONLIN/spring98/human2.htm

Niemi, R.G., & Phillips, J.E. (1980). On nonscience premedical education: Surprising evidence and a call for clarification. *Academic Medicine, 55*, 194-200.

Parsons, T. (1939). The professions and social structure. *Social Forces, 17*, 457-467.

Pellegrino, E. (1974). Educating the humanist physician: An ancient ideal reconsidered. *Journal of the American Medical Association, 227*, 1288-1294.

Porter, R. (1997). *The greatest benefit to mankind: A medical history of humanity.* New York: Norton.

Roche, W.P., Scheetz, A.P., Dane, F.C., Parish, D.C., & O'Shea, J.T. (2003). Medical Students' attitudes in a PBL curriculum: Trust, altruism, and cynicism. *Academic Medicine, 78,* 398-402.

Rodenhauser, P., Strickland, M.A., Gambala, C.T. (2004). Arts-related activities across U.S. medical schools: A follow-up study. *Teaching and Learning in Medicine, 16*(3), 233-239.

Schoen, D. (1987). *Educating the reflective practitioner.* San Francisco, CA: Jossey-Bass.

Shapiro, J., & Rucker, L. (2003). Can poetry make better doctors? Teaching the humanities and arts to medical students and residents at the University of California, Irvine, College of Medicine. *Academic Medicine, 78*, 953-957.

Shapiro, J., Morrison, E.H., & Boker, J.R. (2004). Teaching empathy to first year medical students: Evaluation of an elective literature and medicine course. *Education for Health, 17*(1), 73-84.

Starr, P. (1982). *The transformation of American Medicine.* New York: Basic Books.

Wear, D., & Kuczewski, M.F. (2004). The professionalism movement: Can we pause? *American Journal of Bioethics, 4*(2), 1-10.

Wilensky, H.L. (1964). The professionalization of everybody? *American Journal of Sociology, 70*, 137-158.

Chapter 13

PROFESSIONALISM AND THE HEISENBERG UNCERTAINTY PRINCIPLE

Laura J. Fochtmann
State University of New York at Stony Brook

INTRODUCTION

Within medical education, discussions of professionalism are becoming more complex and simultaneously garnering increased attention (Arnold, 2002; Boon & Turner, 2004; Kao, Lim, Spevick, & Barzansky, 2003; Klein et al., 2003; Ludmerer, 1999; Lynch, Surdyk, & Eiser, 2004; Smith, 2005; Swick, Szenas, Danoff, & Whitcomb, 1999; Swick, 2000; Veloski, Fields, Boex, & Blank, 2005). At the same time, concerns about physician's professional behaviors (Relman, 1998; Morrison & Wickersham, 1998; Kohn, Corrigan, & Donaldson, 2000; Institute of Medicine Committee on Quality of Health Care in America, 2001) are resulting in mandates to assure competency in professionalism (ABIM, 2002; ACGME, 1999; AAMC, 1998). It is in this educational milieu that we must reflect on our approaches to measuring professionalism and the implications of those measurements for students, faculty and patients. The uncertainty principle, which Werner Heisenberg elaborated in 1927, is proposed as a focal point for such reflection.

The Heisenberg Uncertainty Principle is "usually stated in the form: $\Delta x \Delta p_x >= h/4\pi$, where Δx is the uncertainty in the x-coordinate of the particle, Δp_x is the uncertainty in the x-component of the particle's momentum, and h is the Planck constant" (Isaacs, 2000). Alternatively, in non-mathematical terms, it states that "the more precisely the position is determined, the less precisely the momentum is known in this instant, and vice versa" (American Institute of Physics, 2005). Apart from the fact that the professionalism movement is gaining momentum, how can this principle be of any relevance to current discourse on the role of professionalism in medical education?

Many people view the Heisenberg Uncertainty Principle as implying that the act of making a measurement alters the system being measured. Although this view is erroneous from the standpoint of quantum mechanics (Styer, 1996), measurements of professionalism within medical education may be context dependent (Arnold, 2002; Epstein & Hundert, 2002; Fochtmann, 2004; Ginsburg et al., 2000; Hundert, Douglas-Steele, & Bickel, 1996; Swick et al., 1999) or modified by the knowledge that professional behavior is being rated (Holden, 2001; Rees & Shepherd, 2005). Position and momentum, like the specific elements of professionalism, may appear to be discrete and absolute entities. However, in actuality, "the position or momentum of a particle in quantum mechanics is not characterized by a single number, but rather by a continuous function" (Zaarur & Pnini, 1998, p. 58). By the same token, our conceptualizations of professionalism may appear to represent distinct categorical ideals, but in clinical practice these traits are more gradated and impossible to define in absolute terms (Boon et al., 2004; Epstein et al., 2002; Fochtmann, 2004; Ginsburg et al., 2000; Swick, 2000; Van De Camp, Vernooij-Dassen, Grol, & Bottema, 2004). Finally, as the preceding paragraph demonstrates, an emphasis on the detailed mathematics of a particular concept or its measurement can sometimes distract from rather than illuminate its importance to the field as a whole. Such may also be true of our current fixation on measuring professionalism competency in medical education.

Few would question the importance of professional standards of behavior in maintaining the ethical ideals of the medical profession or in fulfilling obligations to patients. In recent years, however, changes in the structure of the health care system and in the delivery of clinical care have been paralleled by changes in physician-patient relationships (ABIM, 2002; Arnold, 2002; Berkman, Wynia, & Churchill, 2004; Castellani & Wear, 2000; Emanuel, Cruess, Cruess, & Hauser, 2002; Ludmerer, 1999; Lundberg, 1991; Relman, 1998; Smith, 2005; Stephenson, Higgs, & Sugarman, 2001; Van Eaton, Horvath, & Pellegrini, 2005). Traditional conceptualizations of professionalism have become more complex. At the same time, concerns about declines in professionalism have been raised in general terms and in association with reports of misconduct by individual physicians (Institute of Medicine Committee on Quality of Health Care in America, 2001; Boon et al., 2004; Kohn et al., 2000; Morrison et al., 1998; Papadakis, Hodgson, Teherani, & Kohatsu, 2004; Relman, 1998; Stern, Frohna, & Gruppen, 2005). In response, professional organizations have delineated more formal standards of professionalism (ABIM, 2002) and credentialing bodies such as the Accreditation Council for Graduate Medical

Education (ACGME) and the Liaison Committee on Medical Education (LCME) have placed an increasing emphasis on the teaching and evaluation of professionalism in all phases of medical education. At face value, it seems entirely reasonable to increase attention to and evaluation of professional behaviors in medical education. Unfortunately, the actual implementation of such initiatives has been less straightforward and has potential pitfalls as well as benefits.

DEFINING PROFESSIONAL BEHAVIOR

Before professionalism can be taught or evaluated, it must first be defined. Behaviors that exemplify professionalism are typically discussed in terms of multiple distinct ideals such as honor, integrity, duty, altruism, respect and accountability (ABIM, 2002; Arnold, 2002; ACGME, 1999; AAMC, 1998; Boon et al., 2004; Epstein et al., 2002; Ginsburg et al., 2000; Ginsburg, Regehr, & Lingard, 2004; Shrank, Reed, & Jernstedt, 2004; Swick, 2000; Van De Camp et al., 2004). However, such ideals are difficult to express in operational terms that lend themselves to teaching or evaluation (Boon et al., 2004; Fochtmann, 2004; Ginsburg et al., 2004; Misch, 2002). Alternatively, professionalism has been viewed in more global and intuitive terms. Misch (2002), for example, has proposed the use of "humanism connoisseurs" to offer a comprehensive judgment of professionalism in the same way that critics would provide an informed opinion on a work of art or musical performance. Others (Gauger, Gruppen, Minter, Colletti, & Stern, 2005) have compared the definition of professionalism to that which Justice Stewart used in describing pornography, "I know it when I see it." Although less well known, Justice Stewart's other remarks on defining obscenity are just as relevant to professionalism when he observed that the courts were "faced with the task of trying to define what may be indefinable" (*Jacobellis v. Ohio,* 1964).

Definitions of professionalism are not absolute

A number of factors contribute to this difficulty in defining professionalism. Although the professional ideals that compose professionalism are typically portrayed in a dichotomous fashion (Fochtmann, 2004; Ginsburg et al., 2000; Misch, 2002; Van De Camp et al., 2004), the related professional behaviors cannot be framed in equally categorical terms. As Gauger et al. (2005) have noted, extreme examples of professional ideals are not necessarily positive. For example, punctuality is a positive trait unless an inordinate amount of time is spent in arriving early to every possible meeting. Professional behaviors may also vary in their frequency of occurrence as well as in the degree to which they exemplify a particular professional ideal (or its opposite). Consequently, if we over generalize from rare events or minor transgressions, erroneous conclusions may be drawn about an individual's professionalism (Fochtmann, 2004). For example, a physician who is habitually rude and disrespectful to patients should be categorized differently in terms of respectfulness than a physician who is typically very courteous but who becomes a bit abrupt with a circumstantial patient fearing that he will be late for surgery. Thus, any valid definitional system should consider such gradations in professional behaviors and not rely solely on absolute definitions of professionalism.

Specific professional behaviors are often interrelated

A related difficulty in delineating and evaluating specific aspects of professionalism is the frequent overlap between professional attributes. Evaluations of physician or student performance can typically be separated into a factor related to technical knowledge and skill and a second factor related to professional and humanistic behaviors (Arnold, 2002; Boon et al., 2004; Dawson-Saunders & Paiva, 1986; Lynch et al., 2004; Maxim & Dielman, 1987; Ramsey et al., 1993; Silber et al., 2004; Veloski et al., 2005). Furthermore, there are often significant correlations between these two factors (Rowley, Baldwin, Jr., Bay, & Cannula, 2000; Herman, Veloski, & Hojat, 1983). Within the realm of professional behaviors, there is also a substantial degree of overlap in specific behaviors. For example, Brownell and Côté (2001) surveyed senior residents about the meaning of professionalism and found that key attributes could be grouped according to expertise/clinical decision-making and doctor-patient relationships/personal qualities. Using factor analysis, Arnold et al. (1998) also found three subcomponents of clinical performance, which were related to excellence, honor/integrity and altruism/respect. Such findings suggest an interdependence of professionalism with other aspects of clinical competence, further complicating the definition and evaluation of professional behavior.

Definitions of professionalism are context dependent

Developing clear-cut operational criteria for judging professional behaviors is made even more difficult by the context-dependent nature of professional interactions (Arnold, 2002; Epstein et al., 2002; Fochtmann, 2004; Ginsburg et al., 2000; Ginsburg, Regehr, Stern, & Lingard, 2002; Ginsburg, Regehr, & Lingard, 2003; Ginsburg et al., 2004; Leach, 2004;

Misch, 2002; Rezler et al., 1992). Of specific ideals of professional behavior, honesty has been most studied. Although physicians vary in their willingness to be deceptive depending upon the context (Ginsburg et al., 2000; Ginsburg et al., 2002; Ginsburg et al., 2004; Green et al., 2000; Novack et al., 1989; Rennie & Crosby, 2001), the vast majority identify some circumstances in which they might engage in deception. The principle of confidentiality is also a hallmark of professionalism but sometimes requires modification depending upon the context. For example, confidentiality may need to be selectively breached to protect the patient or others from imminent harm (American Psychiatric Association, 2001). An additional confound is the fact that perceptions of behavior differ across individuals (Ginsburg et al., 2002; Ginsburg et al., 2004) as well as across clinical and cultural contexts (Misch, 2002).

Specific professional behaviors may conflict with one another

In part because of their context-dependent and interdependent nature, there are often circumstances in which specific professional ideals will come into conflict (Arnold, 2002; Doukas, 2004; Ginsburg et al., 2000; Ginsburg et al., 2004; Jecker, 2004; Klein et al., 2003; Sugarman, 2004; Swick, 2000). For example, as discussed above, in some situations the primacy of the patient's well-being may require an attenuation of confidentiality (American Psychiatric Association, 2001). Under other conditions, the need to protect confidentiality may require some degree of dishonesty (Ginsburg et al., 2000; Novack et al., 1989). While some have decried the negative impact of the hidden curriculum on professional values (Coulehan & Williams, 2001; Hundert, Hafferty, & Christakis, 1996), there are also circumstances in which an excessive emphasis on professional virtues such as empathy or altruism may impair one's ability to provide essential patient care. For example, deferring an indicated lumbar puncture out of empathy for a child's pain would not be in the child's ultimate interest. By the same token, seemingly altruistic behaviors may actually represent boundary violations and diminutions in the physician's objectivity that ultimately have a negative effect on the physician-patient relationship and the patient's clinical outcome (Glass, 2003; Gutheil & Gabbard, 1998; Norris, Gutheil, & Strasburger, 2003). Thus, there are some circumstances in which the hidden curriculum may provide more appropriate context-dependent guidance than the conflicting ideals of the explicit curriculum. At the systems level, professional ideals that reflect the physician's broader commitments to society may come into conflict with duties to individual patients (Swick, 2000). Such conflicts may become increasingly prevalent as financial constraints on medical care continue to worsen (Klein et al., 2003).

TEACHING ABOUT PROFESSIONALISM

From the above, it follows that curricular efforts relating to professionalism need to emphasize the complex gradations and context dependence of professional behaviors as well as the sometimes conflicting nature of professional ideals. In actual practice, however, such an emphasis may not be present. Actual data on the teaching of professionalism comes primarily from surveying medical schools (DuBois & Burkemper, 2002; Kao et al., 2003; Lehmann, Kasoff, Koch, & Federman, 2004; Swick et al., 1999). Such surveys demonstrate a wide degree of variability in the topics and teaching methods used in professionalism related curricula. Typically, much of the explicit instruction occurred in the pre-clinical years and addressed aspects of medical ethics, such as informed consent or confidentiality (DuBois et al., 2002; Kao et al., 2003; Lehmann et al., 2004; Swick et al., 1999). Although many of the surveyed institutions used case-based approaches to learning, either in lectures or small group discussions (DuBois et al., 2002; Kao et al., 2003; Lehmann et al., 2004; Swick et al., 1999), pre-clinical students are not likely to appreciate the nuances of specific clinical scenarios. Many institutions also included training on ethics or professionalism in their clinical clerkships, but developing a cohesive curriculum across diverse clerkships and clerkship sites was viewed as a major challenge (Lehmann et al., 2004).

In contrast to the reported approaches to teaching about ethics or professionalism, students learning about such topics has been said to occur primarily in the clinical years and predominantly through the informal or hidden curriculum (DuBois et al., 2002; Kao et al., 2003; Lehmann et al., 2004; Swick et al., 1999). Although this hidden curriculum has often been described in negative terms as a vehicle for developing cynical and uncaring attitudes, it is clear that informal positive role-modeling can be an equally strong contributor to professional behavior. For example, Brownell and Côté (2001) surveyed 533 senior residents at two Canadian faculties of medicine about characteristics of professionalism and the ways in which professionalism was taught. Of the 258 respondents (response rate 48.4%), more than 90% reported learning about professionalism through positive role models, a figure that was relatively consistent across specialties. Less consistent was the degree to which learning about professionalism occurred through exposure to negative role models, yet this was reported by 28 to 63% of respondents depending upon their sex and medical specialty. In terms of the specific ways in which such role modeling can occur, Barry et al. (2000) surveyed a total of 2207 Colorado medical students, residents and physicians (response rate 44%) on their responses to specific scenarios that represented challenges to professionalism. As part of the survey, respondents were asked about the settings in which they had reviewed similar issues in professionalism. Informal discussions were reported by the majority (76%) as the source of greatest discussion, with about half reporting informal discussion as the source of greatest learning. Interestingly, although only a quarter of respondents described discussing professionalism in teaching rounds or course work and an even fewer number noted these approaches as contributing the most to learning. Teaching rounds were the source of greatest learning for 81% of those who provided a best or acceptable response to the ethical scenarios (Barry et al., 2000). Thus, clinical role modeling has a substantial effect on the learning of professionalism by medical students and residents, regardless of whether such role modeling occurs through informal discussion or during teaching rounds.

In addition to being a common route to learning about professionalism, role modeling may also be the approach that is preferred by trainees. Roberts et al. (2004) surveyed 541 medical students and residents at the University of New Mexico (response rate 62%) on their perceptions of professionalism and ethics education. Regardless of their sex or stage of training, respondents consistently preferred clinically oriented approaches to learning about professionalism, such as role modeling of ethical reasoning and behavior by faculty during clinical rounds, interactions with patients in routine training, and case conferences. Multidisciplinary expertise-oriented learning approaches (e.g., incorporation of ethical issues into lectures, and discussions of cultural aspects of patient care with cultural experts, clinical ethics with ethics consultants, legal aspects with attorneys, and spiritual aspects with chaplains) were also rated highly. Although more typically used in formal curricula, other approaches to learning about professionalism (e.g., peer group discussion led by a knowledgeable clinician, videotapes on ethics followed by discussion led by a knowledgeable clinician, peer group discussions without leadership, interactions with standardized patients, grand rounds presentations, lectures, independent reading, directed reading with tutorial discussions, directed ethics research with a mentor, web-based education) received neutral or only somewhat effective ratings (Roberts et al., 2004). These findings are deserving of replication but suggest a need to reassess more typical curricular approaches to the teaching of professionalism.

EVALUATING PROFESSIONALISM

Regardless of how well we have defined professional behaviors and developed our curricular approaches to professionalism, we must still develop and implement methods for evaluating professionalism in our trainees. Such measures serve a number functions by documenting the competency of students and residents and by conveying that professionalism is an important component of medical education. Consequently, they are being increasingly mandated by accrediting organizations such as the LCME and ACGME (ABIM, 2002; ACGME, 1999; AAMC, 1998).

Specific approaches to the rating of professionalism

In rating professionalism, a number of different approaches have been taken. Although courses in ethics and professionalism may assess student knowledge and performance through written testing or class participation, most evaluation of professionalism is observational in nature. In practice, many ratings are done using Likert scale assessments of multiple different behavioral characteristics (Arnold, 2002; Boon et al., 2004; Lynch et al., 2004; Veloski et al., 2005). Such multidimensional assessments can provide students with feedback on their behavior (Silber et al., 2004), but completion of ratings can be time consuming (Boon et al., 2004). In addition, the rated characteristics are not always continuously distributed (Gauger et al., 2005) or independent of one another (Arnold, 2002; Arnold & Forrow, 1993; Donnelly, Sloan, Plymale, & Schwartz, 2000; Ginsburg et al., 2000; Hodges, Turnbull, Cohen, Bienenstock, & Norman, 1996; Prislin, Lie, Shapiro, Boker, & Radecki, 2001).

Furthermore, the relative nature of such ratings may make it difficult to identify students whose performance is of greatest concern or most in need of remediation. Other evaluation approaches have focused on identifying specific problematic behaviors or rating aspects of professional behavior in more categorical terms (e.g. excellent/solid/concern/problem, meets expectations/needs improvement/cannot assess) (Klein et al., 2003; Larkin, Binder, Houry, & Adams, 2002; Papadakis, Osborn, Cooke, & Healy, 1999; Papadakis, Loeser, & Healy, 2001). Such approaches have the advantage of providing students with specific feedback on professional behaviors and simultaneously identifying those in need of further monitoring or remediation (Papadakis et al., 2001). Global ratings of performance have also been used frequently (Gray, 1996; Littlefield, Paukert, & Schoolfield, 2001; Silber et al., 2004), which may require less time for completion but are less apt to provide trainees with useful feedback (Ende, 1983; Littlefield et al., 2001; Shrank et al., 2004). Although many such scales request narrative elaboration from evaluators, such feedback is often cursory if present at all (Misch, 2002). Detection of problematic behavior may also be less likely with global ratings, since weaknesses in one set of skills may be offset by strong skills in other assessment domains (Hemmer, Hawkins, Jackson, &

Pangaro, 2000; Hunt, 1992; Larkin et al., 2002; Silber et al., 2004; Tonesk, 1983).

Approaches to the rating of professionalism also depend upon the individual who is completing the evaluation, the setting of the evaluation and the timing of the evaluation relative to a given behavior. For example, the majority of evaluations are completed retrospectively, in some instances long after the actual observation of the student's behavior. In other circumstances (e.g. OSCE), evaluation occurs in a concurrent and prospective fashion (Shrank et al., 2004; van Zanten, Boulet, Norcini, & McKinley, 2005). In terms of the evaluative setting, some are naturalistic (e.g., clinical inpatient or ambulatory settings) whereas others are scripted (e.g., OSCE) and at times appear artificial or contrived (Arnold et al., 1993; Ginsburg et al., 2000; Norman et al., 1993; Prislin et al., 1998). In addition to the traditional rating of student performance by faculty, more recent approaches to the rating of professionalism have included self-assessment (Arnold, 2002; Boon et al., 2004; Ginsburg et al., 2000; Lynch et al., 2004; Stern et al., 2005; Veloski et al., 2005) and peer-evaluation (Arnold, 2002; Boon et al., 2004; Gauger et al., 2005; Ginsburg et al., 2000; Lynch et al., 2004; Veloski et al., 2005). More recently, emphasis has been given to the 360 degree or multisource evaluation (ACGME, 1999; Arnold et al., 1998; Larkin et al., 2002; Rees et al., 2005; Rodgers & Manifold, 2002; Shrank et al., 2004; Weigelt, Brasel, Bragg, & Simpson, 2004), in which evaluations are completed by multiple individuals who have come into contact with the student (e.g. other students, residents, faculty, patients, patients' families, nursing staff, other hospital staff). Self-assessment is typically an integral part of the 360 degree evaluation.

Despite this wide variety in approaches to the measurement of professionalism, current evaluative methods are often described as inadequate (ACGME, 1999; Arnold et al., 1998; Murray, Gruppen, Catton, Hays, & Woolliscroft, 2000; Prislin et al., 2001; Shrank et al., 2004; Silber et al., 2004), leading to the suggestion that multiple evaluative approaches should be used (ACGME, 1999; Arnold, 2002; Shrank et al., 2004; van Zanten et al., 2005). Still, the problems with rating professionalism are manifold and may not be resolvable simply by increasing the number of evaluative approaches or evaluations.

PITFALLS IN EVALUATION OF PROFESSIONALISM

Limited reliability of ratings

Given the complexities and context-dependence of professional behavior, it is not surprising that the evaluation of professionalism is limited by the limited reliability of ratings (Arnold, 2002; Boon et al., 2004; Ginsburg et al., 2000; Lynch et al., 2004; Veloski et al., 2005). Studies of 360 degree evaluation show that ratings of medical students are not well correlated (Matthews & Feinstein, 1989; McLeod, Tamblyn, Benaroya, & Snell, 1994; Ramsey et al., 1993; Rees et al., 2005; Weaver, Ow, Walker, & Degenhardt, 1993) and vary significantly depending upon whether the evaluation is completed by a faculty member, a resident, a nurse, or a patient (Arnold, 2002; Johnson & Cujec, 1998). Because inter-rater reliability is often low, multiple assessments are needed to achieve reliable results. The number of assessments can be prohibitive ranging from 10 for ratings by nurses or physicians to as many as 50 for ratings by patients (Ginsburg et al., 2000; Ramsey et al., 1993; Singer, Cohen, Robb, & Rothman, 1993; Singer, Robb, Cohen, Norman, & Turnbull, 1996; Smith, Balint, Krause, Moore-West, & Viles, 1994; Woolliscroft, Howell, Patel, & Swanson, 1994). Even when variations in the clinical scenarios are minimized through the use of OSCEs (Altshuler & Kachur, 2001; Hodges et al., 1996; Klamen & Williams, 1997; Roberts & Norman, 1990; Rogers & Coutts, 2000; Shrank et al., 2004; van Zanten et al., 2005), ratings are dependent upon OSCE content, plus multiple OSCE stations are needed to achieve reliable results (Donnelly et al., 2000; Singer et al., 1993; Singer et al., 1996; Smith et al., 1994).

Yet another impediment to reliable rating is the interconnectedness of professionalism and communication skills. This has been demonstrated with OSCEs (Arnold, 2002; Arnold et al., 1993; Donnelly et al., 2000; Ginsburg et al., 2000; Hodges et al., 1996; Prislin et al., 1998; Prislin et al., 2001) and, as already discussed above, is also likely to be an issue in typical clinical settings. Other errors in ratings may relate to the retrospective nature of evaluations, their tendency to be non-specific (Littlefield et al., 2005) or be influenced by significant halo effects (Arnold, 2002; Gauger et al., 2005; Ginsburg et al., 2000; Misch, 2002; Murden, Way, Hudson, & Westman, 2004; Richards & Wolff, 1982).

Ratings by faculty, peers and others can also be influenced by a variety of biases including sex (Boon et al., 2004; van Zanten et al., 2005; Woolliscroft et al., 1994), race (Boon et al., 2004) and ethnicity (Arnold, 2002; Merrill et al., 1987). When ratings are done by patients, the age and illness of the patient also influences the evaluation (Woolliscroft et al., 1994).

Self-assessments, in particular, are quite inaccurate (Arnold, 2002; Ginsburg et al., 2000; Gordon, 1991; Gordon, 1992; Hodges, Regehr, & Martin, 2001; Jankowski et al., 1991; Linn, Arostegui, & Zeppa, 1975; Stern et al., 2005) and only weakly related to ratings by others (Arnold, Willoughby, & Calkins, 1985; Arnold, 2002; Klessig, Robbins, Wieland, & Rubenstein, 1989; McLeod et al., 1994; Stern et al., 2005). Particularly worrisome is the observation that students who receive lower ratings, presumably reflecting lower competence, overestimate their actual performance (Gordon, 1991; Hodges et al., 2001; Stern et al., 2005).

The fact that egregiously unprofessional behaviors are infrequent can make it difficult to reliably identify professionalism deficiencies (Arnold, 2002). The likelihood that an evaluation will detect a deficiency in professionalism also appears to vary with the setting of the evaluation. For example, on clinical clerkships, problems with professionalism are more likely to be detected during inpatient rotations than during ambulatory care experiences (Gauger et al., 2005; Hemmer et al., 2000). This may relate to variations in the reliability of rating scales in different settings or to the greater workload and degree of stress, greater emphasis on teamwork, and greater continuity of relationships between students and raters on inpatient services (Hemmer et al., 2000). Regardless of the evaluative setting, however, professionalism deficiencies in medical school showed a low sensitivity for predicting future state medical board disciplinary action (Papadakis et al., 2004).

Reliability is also diminished by the fact that physicians often disagree about the delimiters of professional or unprofessional behavior (Ginsburg et al., 2000; Ginsburg et al., 2004; Misch, 2002). Even individual physicians show a considerably degree of inconsistency in the way in which they apply principles of ethics or professionalism (Ginsburg et al., 2004; Green et al., 2000; Novack et al., 1989; Rennie et al., 2001). While these findings speak to the complex and context-dependent nature of professionalism, they also highlight the inherent problems in reliably assessing professionalism across students and clinical settings.

Reluctance of raters to document professional lapses

Even when professional lapses are relatively clear cut, faculty are reluctant to highlight these deficiencies in formal evaluations or discuss these deficiencies verbally with students (Arnold, 2002; Boon et al., 2004; Burack, Irby, Carline, Root, & Larson, 1999; Gauger et al., 2005; Gordon, 1997; Hemmer et al., 2000; Kreiter, Ferguson, Lee, Brennan, & Densen, 1998; Markakis, Beckman, Suchman, & Frankel, 2000; Murden et al., 2004;

Papadakis et al., 1999; Phelan, Obenshain, & Galey, 1993; Rhoton, 1994; Shrank et al., 2004). A reluctance to evaluate attributes of professionalism is not simply limited to faculty evaluations, as many individuals are reluctant to rate themselves (Arnold, 2002; Boon et al., 2004; Gordon, 1991; Gordon, 1992) and peer evaluations are equally difficult to obtain (Arnold, 2002; Helfer, 1972; Shrank et al., 2004; Thomas, Gebo, & Hellmann, 1999; Van Rosendaal & Jennett, 1992). The more subjective nature of professionalism evaluations makes it harder to delineate the specific reasons for a negative evaluation and diminishes rater confidence in their evaluation (Papadakis et al., 1999). In addition, many faculty have already experienced the negative ways in which students respond to feedback (Papadakis et al., 2001), no matter how constructively it may be offered. Those faculty whose academic advancement or salary support is dependent upon teaching evaluations may specifically wish to avoid identifying professionalism deficiencies that may anger students (Burack et al., 1999). Faculty evaluators may also come into conflict with medical school administrators who wish to minimize legal repercussions or student alienation. Thus, for many faculty, a non-response is often the easiest response when confronted by professionalism deficiencies in their students.

Another reason that faculty may avoid rating professional behaviors relates to the dichotomous way in which professionalism is typically defined. As a result, minor behavioral discrepancies from professional ideals may be termed "unprofessional," with all of the potentially harsh consequences of such a label (Burack et al., 1999; Fochtmann, 2004; Gauger et al., 2005; Ginsburg et al., 2000; Stern, 1998). In addition, since grossly unprofessional behaviors are infrequent (Arnold, 2002), typical survey approaches may over-identify professional lapses. For example, a greater apparent rate of professional deficiencies will be found by asking if one has ever observed specific professional lapses without also determining the total number of professional interactions observed (Baldwin, Jr., Daugherty, & Rowley, 1998; Szauter et al., 2003). By the same token, many individuals may have observed or heard about the same serious professional lapse, further inflating the number of reported deficiencies. By potentially over-reporting serious lapses or over-labeling less serious lapses as "unprofessional," recent surveys of professional behaviors may fuel dichotomous conceptualizations and enhance faculty reluctance to rate professionalism.

Ratings of professionalism as burdensome busy work

Despite the essential role of professionalism in medical practice and medical education, faculty often view the rating of professional behaviors as burdensome (Boon et al., 2004; Gauger et al., 2005; Van Luijk, Smeets, Smits, Wolfhagen, & Perquin, 2002). In an era of educational cost containment, evaluative strategies including OSCEs can be expensive in terms of faculty time and direct monetary costs (Gauger et al., 2005). Like many of the other evaluative mandates that have proliferated in recent years, ratings of professionalism are viewed as but another bureaucratic mandate (Anijar, 2004) that has little positive return. In distinguishing between accountability for professional behaviors and accountancy (with a primary emphasis on measurement per se), Anijar (2004) highlights the crux of the issue. Although advocating professional behavior for our students, faculty are much less likely to advocate the detailed and seemingly incessant measurement of such behavior.

There are a number of reasons for this apparent paradox. Faculty members intuitively recognize the poor reliability and multiple other problems with ratings that have been delineated above. While the time required to complete a single evaluation may seem insignificant, many clinical faculty are required to complete multiple evaluations on a significant number of medical students and residents each rotation (typically monthly). With the championing of the 360 degree evaluation, clerkship and residency training directors as well as other faculty members see their administrative burdens as ballooning exponentially for minimal positive return (Weigelt et al., 2004). At times, the use of 360 degree evaluations can even be destructive (Rees et al., 2005; Wimer, 2002). Faculty already perceive that their time with students is too limited or fragmented to effectively engage in teaching (Christakis & Feudtner, 1997; Ginsburg et al., 2000; Papadakis et al., 1999; Papadakis et al., 2001). With the increasing demands to complete ratings of student performance, faculty members are simultaneously confronted by the need to rate students they hardly know and the fact that their limited teaching time is further constrained by time spent on completing evaluations. There is a failure to recognize that faculty members are simply circling numbers to be done with the exercise so they can return to their clinical and educational missions. More worrisome is the fact that inordinate interest in the rating process may actually divert our attention from teaching the underlying principles of professional behavior.

Dealing with the uncertainties of education and evaluation as they relate to professionalism

Like the busy clinician who is required to make medical decisions using imperfect data, medical educators are left with the tasks of teaching and assuring student competence using poorly operationalized and unreliably rated constructs of professional behavior. Fortunately, although the hidden curriculum of medicine's apprenticeship tradition is said to have a negative impact on professionalism, it may also hold clues to solving this conundrum.

Since the organization of medical institutions has traditionally been a strictly hierarchical one, medical leaders (e.g., medical school deans, department chairs, hospital chief executive officers) must first recognize the importance of professionalism to the day-to-day education of students and care of patients as well as to the future of medicine. This step has been achieved to some degree (ABIM, 2002; Cohen, 2004; Institute of Medicine Committee on Quality of Health Care in America, 2001) but many continue to pay lip service to the concepts, focusing instead on collecting sufficient ratings of professional behaviors for their organization's next accreditation visit. If medical leaders address issues of professionalism themselves, faculty and trainees will gradually see such discussions as integral parts of clinical education. Even though published studies suggest that informal discussions or teaching rounds are more effective and more valued in learning about professionalism (Barry et al., 2004; Brownell et al., 2001; Roberts et al., 2004), medical leaders can begin to establish a culture of respect for professionalism teaching through avenues such as grand rounds, clinical case conferences, or morbidity and mortality conferences in which they *themselves* are active participants (Appelbaum & Reiser, 1981).

To maintain credibility with clinical faculty and trainees, however, such educational efforts should use actual clinical scenarios as a springboard for discussion. In addition, rather than relying on free-form discussion or expressions of personal beliefs, a systematic approach should be taken that outlines the specifics of the clinical problem, the precise nature of the ethical dilemma or professionalism issue, and the existing knowledge base (in medicine, law or other fields) that relates to the clinical situation. Insofar as is possible, this approach should parallel that used for other types of clinical decision-making, emphasizing the context-dependent nature of the clinical question. Rather than focusing on superhuman ideals of dichotomously defined professional behaviors, such discussions would encourage students and faculty to strive to improve without setting unrealistic standards of behavioral perfection. This type of educational model would continue to draw upon the expertise of ethicists, philosophers and others, but such individuals would serve as specialty consultants rather than taking on a primary role for education about professionalism.

The second step to enhancing professionalism education requires a willingness to break our addiction to measurement, allowing clinical educators and students to focus their time and efforts on professionalism in the more global sense. It will still be important to highlight significant deficiencies in professional behavior that may presage future unprofessional conduct or harm to patients (Papadakis et al., 1999; Papadakis et al., 2004), but eliminating the need to complete large numbers of minimally informative ratings will abolish most of the problems with evaluation that have been outlined above. In addition, faculty may paradoxically have fewer negative attitudes about focusing on professionalism topics and may have additional time to spend on faculty development and in being more effective role models. Some may argue that less attention to the measurement of professionalism competency may cause students to continue to devalue the important role of professionalism in their education. Although as yet an untested hypothesis, the opposite may actually be true. If combined with a leadership emphasis on professionalism in clinical contexts, students may be able to focus less on trying to fit their behavior to nebulous criteria and begin to grasp and internalize the true meaning of being a professional.

Each of these steps has a common goal of improving the role modeling of professional behaviors by "front-line" clinical educators, which is the lynchpin of learning about professionalism (Branch, Jr. & Paranjape, 2002; Brownell et al., 2001; Ficklin, Browne, Powell, & Carter, 1988; Kenny, Mann, & MacLeod, 2003; Lowenstein, 2003; Ludmerer, 1999; Maheux et al., 2000; Reiser, 1994; Shrank et al., 2004; Wallace, 1997; Wright & Carrese, 2002). Although focusing primarily on the physician-patient relationship and related aspects of professional behaviors, such role modeling can also serve as a starting point for consideration of other aspects of professionalism. For example, enhancing empathy for patients, including those who are disadvantaged, could foster increased social awareness. Rather than encouraging sociopolitical activism that is more in the physician's own interest than in patient interests, social awareness that is rooted in patient encounters is more likely to embody the broader aims of professionalism. Thus, by returning to the traditional models of apprenticeship learning, we can increase faculty and student involvement, address the difficulties in measuring gradated and context-dependent professional behaviors, and work to resolve the growing uncertainties about professionalism education.

REFERENCES

Accreditation Council for Graduate Medical Education (ACGME). (1999). *Outcome project.* Retrieved July 1, 2005 from the website: http://www.acgme.org/outcome/comp/compFull.asp

Altshuler, L., & Kachur, E. (2001). A culture OSCE: Teaching residents to bridge different worlds. *Academic Medicine, 76,* 514.

American Board of Internal Medicine Foundation, ACPBASIM Foundation, and European Federation of Internal Medicine. (2002). Medical professionalism in the new millennium: A physician charter. *Annals of Internal Medicine, 136,* 243-246.

American Institute of Physics. (2005). *Quantum mechanics 1925-1927: The uncertainty principle.* Retrieved on July 1, 2005 from the Website: http://www.aip.org/history/heisenberg/p08.htm

American Psychiatric Association (2003). Practice guideline for the assessment and treatment of patients with suicidal behaviors. *American Journal of Psychiatry, 160,* 1-60.

American Psychiatric Association (2001). *The principles of medical ethics with annotations especially applicable to psychiatry.* Washington, DC: American Psychiatric Publishing.

Anijar, K. (2004). Discourse as rock formation: Fruitcake as professionalism. *American Journal of Bioethics, 4,* W8-10.

Appelbaum, P. S., & Reiser, S. J. (1981). Ethics rounds: A model for teaching ethics in the psychiatric setting. *Hospital and Community Psychiatry, 32,* 555-560.

Arnold, E. L., Blank, L. L., Race, K. E., & Cipparrone, N. (1998). Can professionalism be measured? The development of a scale for use in the medical environment. *Academic Medicine, 73,* 1119-1121.

Arnold, L. (2002). Assessing professional behavior: Yesterday, today, and tomorrow. *Academic Medicine, 77,* 502-515.

Arnold, L., Willoughby, T. L., & Calkins, E. V. (1985). Self-evaluation in undergraduate medical education: A longitudinal perspective. *Journal of Medical Education, 60,* 21-28.

Arnold, R. M., & Forrow, L. (1993). Assessing competence in clinical ethics: Are we measuring the right behaviors. *Journal of General Internal Medicine, 8,* 52-54.

Association of American Medical Colleges (1998). Learning objectives for medical student education: Guidelines for medical schools, medical school objectives project January 1998. Retrieved July 1, 2005, from the Website: http://www.aamc.org/meded/msop/msop1.pdf

Baldwin, D. C., Jr., Daugherty, S. R., & Rowley, B. D. (1998). Unethical and unprofessional conduct observed by residents during their first year of training. *Academic Medicine, 73,* 1195-1200.

Barry, D., Cyran, E., & Anderson, R. J. (2000). Common issues in medical professionalism: Room to grow. *American Journal of Medicine, 108,* 136-142.

Barry, L., Blair, P. G., Cosgrove, E. M., Cruess, R. L., Cruess, S. R., Eastman, A. B. et al. (2004). One year, and counting, after publication of our ACS code of professional conduct. *Journal of American College of Surgeons, 199,* 736-740.

Berkman, N. D., Wynia, M. K., & Churchill, L. R. (2004). Gaps, conflicts, and consensus in the ethics statements of professional associations, medical groups, and health plans. *Journal of Medical Ethics, 30,* 395-401.

Boon, K., & Turner, J. (2004). Ethical and professional conduct of medical students: Review of current assessment measures and controversies. *Journal of Medical Ethics, 30,* 221-226.

Branch, W. T., Jr., & Paranjape, A. (2002). Feedback and reflection: Teaching methods for clinical settings. *Academic Medicine, 77,* 1185-1188.

Brownell, A. K., & Cote, L. (2001). Senior residents' views on the meaning of professionalism and how they learn about it. *Academic Medicine, 76,* 734-737.

Burack, J. H., Irby, D. M., Carline, J. D., Root, R. K., & Larson, E. B. (1999). Teaching compassion and respect: Attending physicians' responses to problematic behaviors. *Journal of General Internal Medicine, 14,* 49-55.

Castellani, B., & Wear, D. (2000). Physician views on practicing professionalism in the corporate age. *Qualitative Health Research, 10,* 490-506.

Christakis, D. A., & Feudtner, C. (1997). Temporary matters: The ethical consequences of transient social relationships in medical training. *Journal of the American Medical Association, 278,* 739-743.

Cohen, J. J. (2004). Ensuring the triumph of professionalism over self-interest. *Association of American Medical Colleges Reporter.* Accessed July 1, 2005 from the Website: http://www.aamc.org/newsroom/reporter/july04/word.htm

Coulehan, J., & Williams, P. C. (2001). Vanquishing virtue: The impact of medical education. *Academic Medicine, 76,* 598-605.

Dawson-Saunders, B., & Paiva, R. E. (1986). Self-evaluation in undergraduate medical education: A longitudinal perspective. *Medical Education, 20,* 240-245.

Donnelly, M. B., Sloan, D., Plymale, M., & Schwartz, R. (2000). Assessment of residents' interpersonal skills by faculty proctors and standardized patients: A psychometric analysis. *Academic Medicine, 75,* S93-S95.

Doukas, D. J. (2004). Returning to professionalism: The re-emergence of medicine's art. *American Journal of Bioethics, 4,* 18-19.

DuBois, J. M., & Burkemper, J. (2002). Ethics education in U.S. medical schools: A study of syllabi. *Academic Medicine, 77,* 432-437.

Emanuel, L., Cruess, R., Cruess, S., & Hauser, J. (2002). Old values, new challenges: What is a professional to do? *International Journal of Qualitative Health Care, 14,* 349-351.

Ende, J. (1983). Feedback in clinical medical education. *Journal of the American Medical Association, 250,* 777-781.

Epstein, R. M., & Hundert, E. M. (2002). Defining and assessing professional competence. *Journal of the American Medical Association, 287,* 226-235.

Ficklin, F. L., Browne, V. L., Powell, R. C., & Carter, J. E. (1988). Faculty and house staff members as role models. *Journal of Medical Education, 63,* 392-396.

Fochtmann, L. J. (2004). The professionalism movement: Pausing and reflecting are essential. *American Journal of Bioethics, 4,* 38-40.

Gauger, P. G., Gruppen, L. D., Minter, R. M., Colletti, L. M., & Stern, D. T. (2005). Initial use of a novel instrument to measure professionalism in surgical residents. *American Journal of Surgery., 189,* 479-487.

Ginsburg, S., Regehr, G., Hatala, R., McNaughton, N., Frohna, A., Hodges, B., et al. (2000). Context, conflict, and resolution: A new conceptual framework for evaluating professionalism. *Academic Medicine, 75,* S6-S11.

Ginsburg, S., Regehr, G., & Lingard, L. (2003). To be and not to be: The paradox of the emerging professional stance. *Medical Education., 37,* 350-357.

Ginsburg, S., Regehr, G., & Lingard, L. (2004). Basing the evaluation of professionalism on observable behaviors: A cautionary tale. *Academic Medicine, 79,* S1-S4.

Ginsburg, S., Regehr, G., Stern, D., & Lingard, L. (2002). The anatomy of the professional lapse: Bridging the gap between traditional frameworks and students' perceptions. *Academic Medicine, 77,* 516-522.

Glass, L. L. (2003). The gray areas of boundary crossings and violations. *American Journal of Psychotherapy, 57,* 429-444.

Gordon, M. J. (1991). A review of the validity and accuracy of self-assessments in health professions training. *Academic Medicine, 66,* 762-769.

Gordon, M. J. (1992). Self-assessment programs and their implications for health professions training. *Academic Medicine, 67,* 672-679.

Gordon, M. J. (1997). Cutting the Gordian knot: A two-part approach to the evaluation and professional development of residents. *Academic Medicine, 72,* 876-880.

Gray, J. D. (1996). Global rating scales in residency education. *Academic Medicine, 71,* S55-S63.

Green, M. J., Farber, N. J., Ubel, P. A., Mauger, D. T., Aboff, B. M., Sosman, J. M., et al. (2000). Lying to each other: When internal medicine residents use deception with their colleagues. *Archives of Internal Medicine, 160,* 2317-2323.

Gutheil, T. G., & Gabbard, G. O. (1998). Misuses and misunderstandings of boundary theory in clinical and regulatory settings. *American Journal of Psychiatry, 155,* 409-414.

Helfer, R. E. (1972). Peer evaluation: Its potential usefulness in medical education. *British Journal of Medical Education, 6,* 224-231.

Hemmer, P. A., Hawkins, R., Jackson, J. L., & Pangaro, L. N. (2000). Assessing how well three evaluation methods detect deficiencies in medical students' professionalism in two settings of an internal medicine clerkship. *Academic Medicine, 75,* 167-173.

Herman, M. W., Veloski, J. J., & Hojat, M. (1983). Validity and importance of low ratings given medical graduates in noncognitive areas. *Journal of Medical Education, 58,* 837-843.

Hodges, B., Regehr, G., & Martin, D. (2001). Difficulties in recognizing one's own incompetence: Novice physicians who are unskilled and unaware of it. *Academic Medicine, 76,* S87-S89.

Hodges, B., Turnbull, J., Cohen, R., Bienenstock, A., & Norman, G. (1996). Evaluating communication skills in the OSCE format: Reliability and generalizability. *Medical Education, 30,* 38-43.

Holden, J. D. (2001). Hawthorne effects and research into professional practice. *Journal of Evaluation in Clinical Practice, 7,* 65-70.

Hundert, E. M., Douglas-Steele, D., & Bickel, J. (1996). Context in medical education: The informal ethics curriculum. *Medical Education, 30,* 353-364.

Hundert, E. M., Hafferty, F., & Christakis, D. (1996). Characteristics of the informal curriculum and trainees' ethical choices. *Academic Medicine, 71,* 624-642.

Hunt, D. D. (1992). Functional and dysfunctional characteristics of the prevailing model of clinical evaluation systems in North American medical schools. *Academic Medicine, 67,* 254-259.

Institute of Medicine Committee on Quality of Health Care in America. (2001). *Crossing the quality chasm: A new health system for the 21st century.* Washington, D.C: National Academy Press.

Isaacs, A. (Ed.) (2000). *A dictionary of physics.* New York: Oxford University Press.

Jankowski, J., Crombie, I., Block, R., Mayet, J., McLay, J., & Struthers, A. D. (1991). Self-assessment of medical knowledge: Do physicians overestimate or underestimate? *Journal of the Royal College of Physicians of London, 25,* 306-308.

Jecker, N. S. (2004). The theory and practice of professionalism. *American Journal of Bioethics, 4,* 47-48.

Johnson, D., & Cujec, B. (1998). Comparison of self, nurse, and physician assessment of residents rotating through an intensive care unit. *Critical Care Medicine, 26,* 1811-1816.

Jacobellis v. Ohio, 378 U.S. 184. (1964). Retrieved July 1, 2005 from the website: http://www.aegis.com/law/SCt/Decisions/1964/378US184.html

Kao, A., Lim, M., Spevick, J., & Barzansky, B. (2003). Teaching and evaluating students' professionalism in U.S. medical schools, 2002-2003. *Journal of the American Medical Association, 290,* 1151-1152.

Kenny, N. P., Mann, K. V., & MacLeod, H. (2003). Role modeling in physicians' professional formation: Reconsidering an essential but untapped educational strategy. *Academic Medicine, 78,* 1203-1210.

Klamen, D. L., & Williams, R. G. (1997). The effect of medical education on students' patient-satisfaction ratings. *Academic Medicine, 72,* 57-61.

Klein, E. J., Jackson, J. C., Kratz, L., Marcuse, E. K., McPhillips, H. A., Shugerman, R. P., et al. (2003). Teaching professionalism to residents. *Academic Medicine, 78,* 26-34.

Klessig, J., Robbins, A. S., Wieland, D., & Rubenstein, L. (1989). Evaluating humanistic attributes of internal medicine residents. *Journal of General Internal Medicine, 4,* 514-521.

Kohn, L. T., Corrigan, J., & Donaldson, M. S. (2000). *To err is human: Building a safer health system.* Washington, D.C: National Academy Press.

Kreiter, C. D., Ferguson, K., Lee, W. C., Brennan, R. L., & Densen, P. (1998). A generalizability study of a new standardized rating form used to evaluate students' clinical clerkship performances. *Academic Medicine, 73,* 1294-1298.

Larkin, G. L., Binder, L., Houry, D., & Adams, J. (2002). Defining and evaluating professionalism: A core competency for graduate emergency medicine education. *Academic Emergency Medicine, 9,* 1249-1256.

Leach, D. C. (2004). Professionalism: The formation of physicians. *American Journal of Bioethics, 4,* 11-12.

Learning objectives for medical student education: Guidelines for medical schools: Report I. of the medical school objectives project. (1999). *Academic Medicine, 74,* 13-18.

Lehmann, L. S., Kasoff, W. S., Koch, P., & Federman, D. D. (2004). A survey of medical ethics education at U.S. and Canadian medical schools. *Academic Medicine, 79,* 682-689.

Linn, B. S., Arostegui, M., & Zeppa, R. (1975). Performance rating scale for peer and self assessment. *British Journal of Medical Education, 9,* 98-101.

Littlefield, J., Paukert, J., & Schoolfield, J. (2001). Quality assurance data for residents' global performance ratings. *Academic Medicine, 76,* S102-S104.

Littlefield, J. H., DaRosa, D. A., Paukert, J., Williams, R. G., Klamen, D. L., & Schoolfield, J. D. (2005). Improving resident performance assessment data: Numeric precision and narrative specificity. *Academic Medicine, 80,* 489-495.

Lowenstein, J. (2003). Where have all the giants gone? Reconciling medical education and the traditions of patient care with limitations on resident work hours. *Perspectives in Biology and Medicine,, 46,* 273-282.

Ludmerer, K. M. (1999). Instilling professionalism in medical education. *Journal of the American Medical Association, 282,* 881-882.

Lundberg, G. D. (1991). Promoting professionalism through self-appraisal in this critical decade. *Journal of the American Medical Association, 265,* 2859.

Lynch, D. C., Surdyk, P. M., & Eiser, A. R. (2004). Assessing professionalism: A review of the literature. *Medical Teacher, 26,* 366-373.

Maheux, B., Beaudoin, C., Berkson, L., Cote, L., Des, M. J., & Jean, P. (2000). Medical faculty as humanistic physicians and teachers: The perceptions of students at innovative and traditional medical schools. *Medical Education, 34,* 630-634.

Markakis, K. M., Beckman, H. B., Suchman, A. L., & Frankel, R. M. (2000). The path to professionalism: Cultivating humanistic values and attitudes in residency training. *Academic Medicine, 75,* 141-150.

Matthews, D. A., & Feinstein, A. R. (1989). A new instrument for patients' ratings of physician performance in the hospital setting. *Journal of General Internal Medicine, 4,* 14-22.

Maxim, B. R., & Dielman, T. E. (1987). Dimensionality, internal consistency and interrater reliability of clinical performance ratings. *Medical Education, 21,* 130-137.

McLeod, P. J., Tamblyn, R., Benaroya, S., & Snell, L. (1994). Faculty ratings of resident humanism predict patient satisfaction ratings in ambulatory medical clinics. *Journal of General Internal Medicine, 9,* 321-326.

Merrill, J. M., Boisaubin, E. V., Jr., Cordova, F. A., Laux, L., Lynch, E. C., Thornby, J. I. et al. (1987). Culture as a determinant of "humanistic traits" in medical residents. *Southern Medical Journal, 80,* 233-236.

Misch, D. A. (2002). Evaluating physicians' professionalism and humanism: the case for humanism connoisseurs. *Academic Medicine, 77,* 489-495.

Morrison, J. & Wickersham, P. (1998). Physicians disciplined by a state medical board. *JAMA, 279,* 1889-1893.

Murden, R. A., Way, D. P., Hudson, A., & Westman, J. A. (2004). Professionalism deficiencies in a first-quarter doctor-patient relationship course predict poor clinical performance in medical school. *Academic Medicine, 79,* S46-S48.

Murray, E., Gruppen, L., Catton, P., Hays, R., & Woolliscroft, J. O. (2000). The accountability of clinical education: Its definition and assessment. *Medical Education, 34,* 871-879.

Norman, G. R., Davis, D. A., Lamb, S., Hanna, E., Caulford, P., & Kaigas, T. (1993). Competency assessment of primary care physicians as part of a peer review program. *Journal of the American Medical Association, 270,* 1046-1051.

Norris, D. M., Gutheil, T. G., & Strasburger, L. H. (2003). This couldn't happen to me: Boundary problems and sexual misconduct in the psychotherapy relationship. *Psychiatric Services, 54,* 517-522.

Novack, D. H., Detering, B. J., Arnold, R., Forrow, L., Ladinsky, M., & Pezzullo, J. C. (1989). Physicians' attitudes toward using deception to resolve difficult ethical problems. *JAMA, 261,* 2980-2985.

Papadakis, M. A., Hodgson, C. S., Teherani, A., & Kohatsu, N. D. (2004). Unprofessional behavior in medical school is associated with subsequent disciplinary action by a state medical board. *Academic Medicine, 79,* 244-249.

Papadakis, M. A., Loeser, H., & Healy, K. (2001). Early detection and evaluation of professionalism deficiencies in medical students: One school's approach. *Academic Medicine, 76,* 1100-1106.

Papadakis, M. A., Osborn, E. H., Cooke, M., & Healy, K. (1999). A strategy for the detection and evaluation of unprofessional behavior in medical students. University of California, San Francisco School of Medicine Clinical Clerkships Operation Committee. *Academic Medicine, 74,* 980-990.

Phelan, S., Obenshain, S. S., & Galey, W. R. (1993). Evaluation of the noncognitive professional traits of medical students. *Academic Medicine, 68,* 799-803.

Prislin, M. D., Fitzpatrick, C. F., Lie, D., Giglio, M., Radecki, S., & Lewis, E. (1998). Use of an objective structured clinical examination in evaluating student performance. *Family Medicine, 30,* 338-344.

Prislin, M. D., Lie, D., Shapiro, J., Boker, J., & Radecki, S. (2001). Using standardized patients to assess medical students' professionalism. *Academic Medicine, 76,* S90-S92.

Ramsey, P. G., Wenrich, M. D., Carline, J. D., Inui, T. S., Larson, E. B., & LoGerfo, J. P. (1993). Use of peer ratings to evaluate physician performance. *Journal of the American Medical Association, 269,* 1655-1660.

Rees, C., & Shepherd, M. (2005). The acceptability of 360-degree judgments as a method of assessing undergraduate medical students' personal and professional behaviours. *Medical Education, 39,* 49-57.

Reiser, S. J. (1994). The ethics of learning and teaching medicine. *Academic Medicine, 69,* 872-876.

Relman, A. S. (1998). Education to defend professional values in the new corporate age. *Academic Medicine, 73,* 1229-1233.

Rennie, S. C., & Crosby, J. R. (2001). Are "tomorrow's doctors" honest? Questionnaire study exploring medical students' attitudes and reported behaviour on academic misconduct. *British Medical Journal, 322,* 274-275.

Rezler, A. G., Schwartz, R. L., Obenshain, S. S., Lambert, P., Gibson, J. M., & Bennahum, D. A. (1992). Assessment of ethical decisions and values. *Medical Education, 26,* 7-16.

Rhoton, M. F. (1994). Professionalism and clinical excellence among anesthesiology residents. *Academic Medicine, 69,* 313-315.

Richards, R. W., & Wolff, H. J. (1982). Measuring the unmeasurable. *Journal of the American Osteopathic Association, 82,* 124-128.

Roberts, J., & Norman, G. (1990). Reliability and learning from the objective structured clinical examination. *Medical Education, 24,* 219-223.

Roberts, L. W., Green Hammond, K. A., Geppert, C. M., & Warner, T. D. (2004). The positive role of professionalism and ethics training in medical education: A comparison of medical student and resident perspectives. *Academic Psychiatry, 28,* 170-182.

Rodgers, K. G., & Manifold, C. (2002). 360-degree feedback: Possibilities for assessment of the ACGME core competencies for emergency medicine residents. *Academic Emergency Medicine, 9,* 1300-1304.

Rogers, J. C. & Coutts, L. (2000). Do students' attitudes during preclinical years predict their humanism as clerkship students? *Academic Medicine, 75,* S74-S77.

Rowley, B. D., Baldwin, D. C., Jr., Bay, R. C., & Cannula, M. (2000). Can professional values be taught? A look at residency training. *Clinical Orthopaedics and Related Research, 378,* 110-114.

Shrank, W. H., Reed, V. A., & Jernstedt, G. C. (2004). Fostering professionalism in medical education: A call for improved assessment and meaningful incentives. *Journal of General Internal Medicine, 19,* 887-892.

Silber, C. G., Nasca, T. J., Paskin, D. L., Eiger, G., Robeson, M., & Veloski, J. J. (2004). Do global rating forms enable program directors to assess the ACGME competencies? *Academic Medicine, 79,* 549-556.

Singer, P. A., Cohen, R., Robb, A., & Rothman, A. (1993). The ethics objective structured clinical examination. *Journal of General Internal Medicine, 8,* 23-28.

Singer, P. A., Robb, A., Cohen, R., Norman, G., & Turnbull, J. (1996). Performance-based assessment of clinical ethics using an objective structured clinical examination. *Academic Medicine, 71,* 495-498.

Smith, L. G. (2005). Medical professionalism and the generation gap. *American Journal of Medicine, 118,* 439-442.

Smith, S. R., Balint, J. A., Krause, K. C., Moore-West, M., & Viles, P. H. (1994). Performance-based assessment of moral reasoning and ethical judgment among medical students. *Academic Medicine, 69,* 381-386.

Stephenson, A., Higgs, R., & Sugarman, J. (2001). Teaching professional development in medical schools. *Lancet, 357,* 867-870.

Stern, D. T. (1998). Practicing what we preach? An analysis of the curriculum of values in medical education. *American Journal of Medicine, 104,* 569-575.

Stern, D. T., Frohna, A. Z., & Gruppen, L. D. (2005). The prediction of professional behaviour. *Medical Education, 39,* 75-82.

Styer, D. F. (1996). Common misconceptions regarding quantum mechanics. *American Journal of Physics, 64,* 31-34.

Sugarman, J. (2004). Pausing to consider recommendations for recasting the professionalism movement in academic medicine. *American Journal of Bioethics, 4,* 16-17.

Swick, H. M. (2000). Toward a normative definition of medical professionalism. *Academic Medicine, 75,* 612-616.

Swick, H. M., Szenas, P., Danoff, D., & Whitcomb, M. E. (1999). Teaching professionalism in undergraduate medical education. *Journal of the American Medical Association, 282,* 830-832.

Szauter, K., Williams, B., Ainsworth, M. A., Callaway, M., Bulik, R., & Camp, M. G. (2003). Student perceptions of professional behavior of faculty physicians. *Medical Education Online, 8,* 17.

Thomas, P. A., Gebo, K. A., & Hellmann, D. B. (1999). A pilot study of peer review in residency training. *Journal of General Internal Medicine, 14,* 551-554.

Tonesk, X. (1983). Clinical judgment of faculties in the evaluation of clerks. *Journal of Medical Education, 58,* 213-214.

Van De Camp, K., Vernooij-Dassen, M. J., Grol, R. P., & Bottema, B. J. (2004). How to conceptualize professionalism: A qualitative study. *Medical Teacher, 26,* 696-702.

Van Eaton, E. G., Horvath, K. D., & Pellegrini, C. A. (2005). Professionalism and the shift mentality: How to reconcile patient ownership with limited work hours. *Archives of Surgery, 140,* 230-235.

Van Luijk, S. J., Smeets, J. G. E., Smits, J., Wolfhagen, I., & Perquin, M. L. F. (2002). Assessing professional behaviour and the role of academic advice at the Maastricht Medical School. *Medical Teacher, 22,* 168-172.

Van Rosendaal, G. M., & Jennett, P. A. (1992). Resistance to peer evaluation in an internal medicine residency. *Academic Medicine, 67,* 63.

van Zanten, M., Boulet, J. R., Norcini, J. J., & McKinley, D. (2005). Using a standardised patient assessment to measure professional attributes. *Medical Education, 39,* 20-29.

Veloski, J. J., Fields, S. K., Boex, J. R., & Blank, L. L. (2005). Measuring professionalism: A review of studies with instruments reported in the literature between 1982 and 2002. *Academic Medicine, 80,* 366-370.

Wallace, A. G. (1997). Educating tomorrow's doctors: The thing that really matters is that we care. *Academic Medicine, 72,* 253-258.

Weaver, M. J., Ow, C. L., Walker, D. J., & Degenhardt, E. F. (1993). A questionnaire for patients' evaluations of their physicians' humanistic behaviors. *Journal of General Internal Medicine, 8,* 135-139.

Weigelt, J. A., Brasel, K. J., Bragg, D., & Simpson, D. (2004). The 360-degree evaluation: Increased work with little return? *Current Surgery, 61,* 616-626.

Wimer, S. (2002). The dark side of 360-degree feedback. *Training and Development 56*(9), 37-41.

Woolliscroft, J. O., Howell, J. D., Patel, B. P., & Swanson, D. B. (1994). Resident-patient interactions: The humanistic qualities of internal medicine residents assessed by patients, attending physicians, program supervisors, and nurses. *Academic Medicine, 69,* 216-224.

Wright, S. M., & Carrese, J. A. (2002). Excellence in role modeling: Insight and perspectives from the pros. *Canadian Medical Association Journal, 167,* 638-643.

Zaarur, E., & Pnini, R. (1998). *Schaum's Outline of Quantum Mechanics.* New York: McGraw Hill.

CODA

David C. Leach
Accreditation Council of Graduate Medical Education

> *The true professional is one who does not obscure grace with illusions of technical prowess, but one who strips away all illusions to reveal a reliable truth in which the human heart can rest.*
>
> Parker J. Palmer, *The Active Life* (1990)

The preceding chapters constitute a major and welcomed intellectual effort to understand, teach and assess medical professionalism. Each chapter adds significantly to the understanding of professionalism; some clarify the concepts of professionalism; some make specific recommendations about the curriculum, others assessment; and some focus on the context in which professionalism is taught. This is a very useful book. While the work speaks for itself, three questions bear repeated emphasis: to what extent is professionalism a social construct; what is the role of individual virtue in attaining professionalism; and how can institutions enable or disable professionalism? A fourth, and I believe unifying, question or theme derives from the above quotation: does the profession obscure truth with illusion or does it strip away illusion to reveal truth?

While I acknowledge that the assumptions of postmodernism and post-structuralism undergird modern society, I still get hives at the very thought of the movement. Thirty years of practicing medicine make it very difficult for me to accept that reality is nothing more than a social construct. In fact I would suggest that medicine offers society relief by approaching truth through classical critical realism (not the anemic early 20th century version of critical realism, but the version going back to Aristotle). An analogy may help explain my bias: I may or may not have a gallstone. If I do, it is not a social construct; I either have it or not and my doctor either diagnoses it correctly or not. But it is a real gallstone. If one hundred doctors say I do not have a gallstone and I do, I do. The approach to the diagnosis and treatment of disease is helped by critical realism. The postmodernist approach takes us back to the dark days of medicine and is rejected.

Some comfort is offered by Lewis' statement that "postmodern philosophy argues *both* that there is a real world *and* that the real world is sufficiently complex to support multiple social constructions that can meaningfully and practically organize it." He argues that "institutional medicine" (a social construct) is the enemy of "medical professionalism" (as aspired to by individual physicians). The resolution of this conflict may consist in recognizing that all institutions are an illusion; the only things real in them are the people and the relationships they have with one another. The "goodness" of professionalism comes from individual professionals making individual decisions to respond to their vocation seriously.

While postmodernism may make a bad master, it can be a good servant. Shirley and Padgett enhance our understanding of the illusions of professionalism by pointing out that the ambiguity of the language "works to unify and solidify social networks and interest," making that unity seem natural. In other words, everyone understands the words being used but they mean something different for each (Hock, 2005). They also, correctly and importantly in my view, point out that the "new professionalism" tends to ignore major social and institutional changes that have important enabling or disabling effects on individual virtue. As the various communities of medicine construct language in an effort to make sense out of phenomena associated with their work, their language surrounding professionalism tends to become context-specific, confounding measurement and communication. Continuing to use the language of professionalism without clarifying its relationship to context and the actual practices seen in daily work confuses all (including trainees) and nurtures hostility; anchoring the abstract in the concrete does the reverse. It is interesting that the first two years of medical school are frequently described as a "giant vocabulary lesson"; students spend an inordinate amount of time getting the language right for the science of disease biology and yet very little time getting the language right for professionalism.

Castellani and Hafferty further the conversation substantially by clarifying the complexities of professionalism and naming its clusters. They give us a basic understanding of professionalism as a complex system and identify it as a way of organizing the work of medicine. Competing elements are identified and specific interventions for researchers, educators and learners are recommended. Their approach is very useful, and yet also depends on a postmodernist framework: complex adaptive systems are designed to make sense out of phenomena and are an example of how to use postmodernism as a servant rather than a master.

As useful as the various social constructs of professionalism are, my own bias is that at its heart professionalism is determined by individual responses to vocation. It is about character development. The work of medicine is such that it is impossible to do without being shaped by it. Professional formation and the quality of patient care are inexorably linked. However, it is daunting to understand the role of individual accountability and the role of the context in which the work is done. It is especially daunting to deconstruct the phenomena enough to teach and measure it. Several chapters in this book address this issue. Inui et al. offer a model that attempts to address the linkage between personal and professional development and to make explicit several examples within the institution that can be used to further this end. The power of the stories in their chapter clarifies the nexus of personal and organizational development. Aultman clarifies the boundaries between ethics and professionalism as a way of enhancing curricular design. Coulehan describes the flaws of teaching virtue in systems hostile to virtues; he uses the words conversion and witnessing, role modeling, self-awareness, community service and narrative competence to get us beyond that difficulty. Wear offers the powerful example of "a pedagogy of discomfort" as a model of teaching both respect for patients and deepening individual self awareness of respect as a key concept of professionalism. The discomfort itself makes the hidden curriculum visible. George et al. offer a specific curricular model based in part on the work of Rachel Remen and soon to be implemented at Case Western that bridges the particular patient-doctor and society-profession aspects of professional relationships. The role of regulators and a possible curricular response to those challenges is offered by Doukas. Fochtmann guides us through the complexities encountered in assessing professionalism and uses apt comparisons with the Heisenberg Uncertainty Principle. All of these chapters offer practical approaches that will be of great interest to those charged with doing this work.

There is, however, a price to be paid for the deconstruction of professionalism. Kuczewski points out that the demand for objective assessment of professionalism may itself narrow and inhibit professional formation. He guides us back to the use of exemplars and paradigms of virtuous development. His definition of professionalism as "the norms that guide the relationships in which physicians engage in the care of patients" gives primacy to the patient and orders the conversation and potential measures in ways that are really helpful. Professionalism is about relationships; it is in relationship that professionals are formed. As Brincat reminds us, without patients, professionalism is meaningless. She also names compassion as its heart. What types of institutions provide guidance to developing professionals about how to nurture compassion in very complex situations?

All of the authors acknowledge what I call the Abraham Verghese problem. Dr. Verghese, at a recent forum convened by the American Board of Internal Medicine (ABIM) and in response to a group celebration of the Physician Charter which details elements of professionalism, brought silence to the group by pointing out (to paraphrase): It is interesting that we pay extraordinary attention to the words used to express our values. Perhaps we do this because they would not otherwise be evident (2005). He noted that when he presents the Physician Charter to medical students they see it as a no-brainer—of course these are the values we should have, that is what drew us into medicine. Yet, these same students then go on a journey to, and only occasionally through, cynicism as they encounter the values of the profession as expressed in the daily work of physicians. It would be immensely helpful to know what types of relationships facilitate and what types inhibit professional formation. What approaches can be taken to incorporate the reality that doctor patient relationships are now housed in and deeply influenced by complex sets of communities, each with competing values and views of goodness? What can be done to root out cynicism? How can developing professionals encounter ever deepening and more meaningful experiences of professionalism rather than the diminishing and isolating experiences now extant? At a time when medicine can do more than ever before, why do we feel so bad?

Let's use Parker Palmer's idea that true professionals strip away illusions to reveal truth as a guide. Oh my! Might that mean that institutions ought to tell the truth about their health care outcomes? Would that mean that they systematically disclose errors, apologize and work diligently to improve health care? Would that mean that advertising budgets would be cut in order to improve rather than disguise the truth? Merton used to say that we exhaust ourselves supporting our illusions (1988). Perhaps students become cynical because they and their mentors are exhausted from supporting illusions. Academic medical centers may be more prone to this than most; not only do they have to do the work of medicine, but they also have to support the set of illusions associated with being academic. We could do worse than to pick as our North Star the task of stripping away illusions to reveal the truth. After all, at a very fundamental level we are all programmed to seek truth, goodness and beauty. Our intellect, will and imagination are designed to do just that, and we might be well-served to work with rather than against nature.

REFERENCES

Palmer, P. (1990). *The active life*. San Francisco: Jossey-Bass.

Hock, D. (July 28, 2005). Personal communication. Olympia, Washington. Dee Hock captured the essence of postmodernism with this expression in a private conversation at this meeting.

Verghese, A. (August 9, 2005). American Board of Internal Medicine Summer Forum, Sun River, Oregon.

Merton, T. (1988). *The true and false self*. Kansas City, MO: Credence Cassettes.

LIST OF CONTRIBUTORS

Julie M. Aultman, Ph.D., received her doctorate in philosophy at Michigan State University and is currently an Assistant Professor at Northeastern Ohio Universities College of Medicine. Her primary research involves both theoretical and pragmatic investigations into the concepts of health and disease, namely mental health, and ethical issues surrounding community-based rehabilitation, treatment adherence, and the use of classification systems in medical practice. Other research areas include the evaluation of teaching practices and curriculum development within medical education, e.g., teaching philosophy to medical students, the role of medical ethics in the clinical setting, and the involvement of humanities within a medical curriculum. Aultman has published and presented her research nationally and internationally.

Cynthia Brincat, M.D., Ph.D., is a graduate of Smith College and received her Ph.D. in philosophy from Loyola University, Chicago. After teaching philosophy and medical ethics for several years she decided to return to Loyola for her M.D. She is presently in her second year of residency in obstetrics and gynecology at the University of Michigan. There she works to integrate her past life into work on informed consent and women's health as well as professionalism in health care. Currently, Brincat can be found every fourth night on the busy labor and delivery unit of the University of Michigan's Women's Birth Center. In between, she brings her theoretical background to empirical research on the impact of cesarean sections over vaginal deliveries, the reaction of the health care establishment as well as the long and short term outcomes to women and their infants.

Brian Castellani, Ph.D., is an Assistant Professor of Sociology at Kent State University. His doctorate is in medical sociology and his Masters is in clinical psychology. Since the publication of his book, *Pathological Gambling* (2000), he has been developing a program of research in the sociology of complexity and is currently completing a monograph on the topic with his colleague Fred Hafferty.

Ann Cottingham M.A.R.., M.A., is a graduate of Duke University, Yale Divinity School and the University of Notre Dame and holds degrees in Literature, Ethics and Theology. She is currently working in medical education at Indiana University School of Medicine in the areas of curricular and organizational development. Cottingham seeks to further develop and expand the formal competency based-curriculum and to improve the learning environment of the informal curriculum.

Jack Coulehan, M.D., is the Director of the Institute for Medicine in Contemporary Society and Professor of Medicine and Preventive Medicine at the State University of New York at Stony Brook. He is the author of four collections of poetry, including *Medicine Stone* (2002), and has authored or edited several other books. The 5th edition of *The Medical Interview: Mastering Skills for Clinical Practice* (F.A. Davis Company, 2005), a best selling text on the clinician-patient relationship; and *Second Opinion*, an anthology of poems by physicians (University of Iowa, 2006) are the most recent. Jack's honors and awards include fellowships from the Pennsylvania Council for the Arts (1988) and National Endowment for the Humanities (1989); the American College of Physicians Poetry Award (1997), the American Nurses Association's award for best book (1998), the Merck Fellowship at Yaddo (1999); and the American Academy of Hospice and Palliative Medicine award for distinction in the humanities (2004).

David John Doukas, M.D., is the William Ray Moore Endowed Chair of Family Medicine and Medical Humanism, and Professor of Family and Geriatric Medicine and of the Institute for Bioethics, Health Policy and Law at the University of Louisville. Doukas is also the Director of the Program for Education in Humanism, Ethics, and Professionalism and also currently serves as Chair of the University of Louisville Hospital Ethics Committee. His degrees include a B.A. in Biology and Religious Studies from the University of Virginia and an M.D. from Georgetown University School of Medicine. After his Family Practice residency at the University of Kentucky, Doukas completed a Post-Doctoral Fellowship in Bioethics (1986-87) at the Joseph and Rose Kennedy Institute of Ethics at Georgetown University and the Franklin Square Hospital Center. Doukas has written extensively on the ethical implications of patient and physician value judgments in the informed consent process. Most recently, he has written on the need to better articulate and integrate educational activities in medical school and residency programs to promote humanism, ethics, and professionalism in medical care.

Danny George, B.A., is a graduate of the College of Wooster and is currently pursuing a master's degree in public health at Case Western Reserve University, while working as a research assistant at the Memory and Aging Center at Case Western Reserve University. His senior thesis, "Can Narrative Heal?" weighs both the merits of narrative-based pedagogy in medical schools and the benefits of narrative therapy story-telling sessions for individuals with dementia. He is currently co-authoring a book entitled *The End of Alzheimer's Disease* with Dr. Peter Whitehouse.

Laura Fochtmann, M.D., is a graduate of Washington University's School of Engineering and School of Medicine. She completed her psychiatry residency at the Johns Hopkins Hospital followed by fellowship training at the National Institutes of Health. Fochtmann is currently Professor of Psychiatry and Behavioral Sciences at Stony Brook University School of Medicine and holds joint appointments in the Departments of Pharmacological Sciences and Emergency Medicine. In addition, she directs the Electroconvulsive Therapy Service at Stony Brook University Hospital and serves as Medical Editor for the American Psychiatric Association Practice Guidelines. Her interests in the teaching and evaluation of professionalism are an outgrowth of her extensive involvement in medical student and resident teaching, which spans clinical as well as didactic settings.

Richard M. Frankel, Ph.D., is Professor of Medicine and Geriatrics and a Senior Research Scientist at the Regenstrief Institute, Indiana University School of Medicine. He is also a senior scientist in the Health Services Unit at the Richard L. Roudebush VAMC. After receiving his Ph.D. in 1977 in medical sociology at the Graduate School and University Center of the City University of New York, Frankel did a post-doctoral fellowship in qualitative approaches to mental health research at Boston University. His research interests include: the physician patient relationship and its effect on the processes and outcomes of care, psychosocial aspects of medical care, communication between older adults and their providers, the effects of technology (computers) on the physician patient relationship, patient safety and communicating about medical errors, and conversations at the end of life. He has published more than 125 scientific papers on these topics.

Iahn Gonsenhauser, B.A., is a research assistant in the Integrative Studies Department at Case Western Reserve University. He attended Syracuse University where he received his B.A. in Psychology. Currently, he is a student of the Weatherhead School of Management's Bioscience Entrepreneurship program. His research focus is on quality of life valuation and decision making in patients with dementia, as well as the effectiveness of volunteering as an intervention to promote healthy aging. His former work can be found in the *Journal of Applied Physiology.*

Frederic W. Hafferty, Ph.D., is Professor of Behavioral Sciences at the University of Minnesota-Duluth, School of Medicine. He received his undergraduate degree in Social Relations from Harvard in 1969 and his Ph.D. in Medical Sociology from Yale in 1976. He is the author of *Into the Valley: Death and the Socialization of Medical Students* (Yale University Press 1991), and co-authored *The Changing Medical Profession: An International Perspective* (Oxford University Press 1993) with John McKinlay. He is currently working on two books: the first (with Al Imershein) is on the role of the stock market in the rise of managed care, and the second is on the hidden curriculum in medical education. He is past chair of the Medical Sociology Section of the American Sociological Association and currently sits on the Association of American Medical College's Council of Academic Societies. Current research focuses on the disappearance of altruism as a core medical value and the concurrent rise of "lifestyle medicine," the role of trust in the ideology of professionalism, social dimensions of medical effectiveness research, disability studies, and rural health issues.

Thomas S. Inui, Sc.M., M.D., is President and CEO of the Regenstrief Institute for Health Care, Inc., the Sam Regenstrief Professor of Health Services Research, and Associate Dean for Health Care Research at Indiana University School of Medicine. Inui is a primary care physician, educator, and researcher. His previous positions include: head of general internal medicine at the University of Washington School of Medicine, and the Paul C. Cabot Professor and the founding chair of the Department of Ambulatory Care and Prevention at Harvard Medical School. Inui's teaching and research emphasizes physician-patient communication, health promotion and disease prevention, the social context of medicine, and medical humanities. He is the author of 245 publications, including the AAMC monograph *A Flag in the Wind: Educating for Professionalism in Medicine* (AAMC, Washington D.C. 2003).

Audiey Kao, M.D., Ph.D. is Vice President of the Ethics Group at the American Medical Association. In this position, Kao oversees the wide array of educational, research, and policy-setting activities relevant to ethics and professionalism. Graduated *magna cum laude* from the University of California at Berkeley with degrees in biochemistry and economics, he received his medical degree from the University of Pennsylvania School of Medicine, and completed his residency training in internal medicine at the Hospital of the University of Pennsylvania. Kao received his doctorate in Health Policy from Harvard University. His dissertation thesis, "Trust and Agency: The Patient-Physician Relationship in the Era of Managed Care," examined the impact of financial incentives on patients' trust in their physicians. His work has been published in *JAMA, New England Journal of Medicine, Academic Medicine*, and other leading medical journals. Kao has been a Visiting Scholar at the Center for Bioethics at the University of Pennsylvania, and has taught at the University of Chicago and the University of Illinois at Chicago. He continues to practice medicine in a volunteer-based free clinic.

Mark G. Kuczewski, Ph.D., is the Father Michael I. English, S.J. Professor of Medical Ethics and the Director of the Neiswanger Institute for Bioethics and Health Policy, Stritch School of Medicine, Loyola University Chicago. He is a philosopher by training whose research and writings have focused extensively on clinical ethical decision making. He is the author of several books including (with Rosa Lynn Pinkus) *An Ethics Casebook for Hospitals: Practical Approaches to Everyday Cases* (Georgetown University Press, 1999). He has written extensively on the teaching of professionalism in medicine, especially fostering a concern for social justice as an aspect of professionalism.

David C. Leach, M.D., is Executive Director of the Accreditation Council for Graduate Medical Education. He received a BA from the University of Toronto in 1965 and an M.D. from the University of Rochester School of Medicine and Dentistry in 1969. He completed residency training in internal medicine and endocrinology at the Henry Ford Health System in Detroit. He was awarded the "Good Samaritan Award" by Governor John Engler for his work over 25 years at a Free Clinic in Detroit. He became interested in medical education and was assistant dean at the University of Michigan for several years, primarily directing the Henry Ford experiences for Michigan students. Dr. Leach then was appointed director of medical education at Henry Ford, and subsequently played a role in the affiliation between Case Western Reserve University School of Medicine and Henry Ford.

Bradley Lewis, M.D., Ph.D., combined his medical and psychiatric training with a study of humanities and social theory. He currently teaches at the interface of medicine, culture, and humanities at New York University's Gallatin School for Individualized Study and at NYU's Psychiatry Department. He is the cultural studies editor for the *Journal of Medical Humanities* and his book, *Moving Beyond Prozac, DSM, and the New Psychiatry: The Birth of Postpsychiatry,* will be published in 2006. His interest in medical professionalism comes from his continued practice of psychiatry and his work mentoring pre-med students and residents.

Debra Litzelman, M.A., M.D., is the Associate Dean for Medical Education and Curricular Affairs at the Indiana University School of Medicine (IUSM) where she teaches clinical medicine and practices as a general internist. She has a Master's degree in Psychology from the University of Southern California. She has combined her interest in primary care medicine and the behavioral sciences to advance the competency based curriculum at IUSM which emphasizes the comprehensive training of knowledgeable and compassionate physicians. Litzelman's publications focus on clinical teaching effectiveness, including the teaching of caring attitudes. She has contributed chapters to the *Guidebook for Clerkship Directors* (2001, 2005) published by the Association of American Medical Colleges.

David L. Mossbarger, M.B.A., M.A., is Project Manager for the Relationship-Centered Care Initiative at Indiana University School of Medicine. He received his B.S. from West Point Military Academy, his M.A. from Ball State University, and his M.B.A. in Management from Indiana University. As a career Army officer, Mossbarger combines his theoretical background with practical experience in the study of organizational behavior. He has taught various college-level business courses to include organizational behavior, management, leadership, and professional development. He joined Regenstrief Institute in 2003.

Stephen M. Padgett, RN, MS, is a doctoral candidate at the University of Washington in the School of Nursing. He has worked as a staff nurse in the fields of acute-care adult medicine, mental health, and home care. His dissertation research is on the sociology of professions, focusing on everyday professional relationships and the negotiation of standards. More broadly, he is interested in health policy and politics, the relationship of language and experience, and the role of gender in divisions of labor and knowledge. He has published several articles on nursing research and the organization of clinical practice.

Jennifer A. Reenan, M.D., is a Senior Research Associate at the American Medical Association. She graduated from the University of Michigan Medical School in 2003 and holds an A.B. in History and Literature from Harvard University. Since 2003, Reenan has worked for the Ethics Standards Group at the American Medical Association, initially in the Institute for Ethics and now in the Office of the Vice President for Ethics where she is currently involved in efforts to develop a national consortium of educators and clinicians interested in medical professionalism and medical education outcomes research. She has also written for the AMA's Virtual Mentor, a journal on ethics for medical students, residents and young physicians.

Jamie L. Shirley, RN, PhD, is a post-doctoral fellow at the Center for Women's Health and Gender Disparities in the School of Nursing at the University of Washington. Her current research examines how practices of autonomy are negotiated within families between caregivers and those for whom they provide care. She recently completed her dissertation, *Autonomy at the End-of-Life: A Discourse Analysis,* at the University of Washington. She teaches ethics to nurses returning to complete their bachelor's degrees at the University of Washington at Tacoma. Her academic work is informed by her clinical experience in home care hospice settings.

Anthony L. Suchman, M.D., M.A., is a practicing internist, Clinical Professor of Medicine and Psychiatry at the University of Rochester, and a consultant to health care organizations on clinical and administrative processes and culture change. He studied medicine at Cornell University, completed a medicine residency and fellowship in General Internal Medicine and Behavioral and Psychosocial Medicine at the University of Rochester. Suchman earned an M.A. in Organizational Change at the University of Hertfordshire's Complexity and Management Centre. Through his teaching and writing he has become known as a leading proponent of the partnership-based clinical philosophy known as Relationship-Centered Care, and now focuses on the application of these principles and practices in the realm of administration and organizational behavior.

T. Robert Vu, M.D., received his B.S. degree from the University of Maryland, College Park, and his medical degree from the University of Maryland School Of Medicine in Baltimore, MD. He did all of his post-graduate training at Indiana University School of Medicine where he is now assistant professor of clinical medicine and serves as director of the internal medicine clerkships. His main areas of teaching and research interests include clinical teaching, faculty development in and evaluation of clinical teaching effectiveness, curriculum development and evaluation, and mindful/reflective practice. He is co-author of a recent ABIM Foundation monograph *Putting the Physician Charter into Practice in Medical School Departments of Medicine.*

Delese Wear, PhD, is Professor of Behavioral Sciences at the Northeastern Ohio Universities College of Medicine where she teaches literature and medicine in the Human Values in Medicine program. She is author of *Privilege in the Medical Academy: A Feminist Examines Gender, Race & Power* (1997) and co-editor (with Janet Bickel) of *Educating for Professionalism: Creating a Climate of Humanism in Medical Education* (2000). In addition to professionalism, her research focuses on teaching and curricular issues in the medical humanities.

Peter J. Whitehouse, MD, PhD is Director of the Integrative Studies at Case Western Reserve University in the Department of Neurology as well as Professor of Cognitive Science, Psychiatry, Neuroscience, Psychology, Nursing, Organizational Behavior and History. He received his undergraduate degree from Brown University and MD-PhD (Psychology) from The Johns Hopkins University, followed by a Fellowship in Neuroscience and Psychiatry and a faculty appointment at Hopkins. In 1986 he founded the University Alzheimer Center at Case Western Reserve University and University Hospitals of Cleveland. He continued his own life-long learning with a Masters Degree in Bioethics and Fellowship in Organizational Behavior at Case. Whitehouse is clinically active at University Hospitals of Cleveland in the Joseph Foley Elder Health Center at Fairhill Center caring for individuals with concerns about their cognitive abilities as they age. He is working to develop an integrative health practice focused on the healing power of story telling. His current NIH grants focus on quality of life, ethics and genetic testing in dementia.

Penny Williamson, Sc.D., is a facilitator, organizational consultant, educator, and coach. She received her doctorate from the Johns Hopkins University, where she teaches physicians communication and teaching skills as an Associate Professor of Medicine. In her independent consulting practice, Williamson facilitates renewal retreats focused on how to find and sustain meaning, spirit, courage, and heart in one's life and work; coaches leaders to enhance their personal and professional effectiveness; and helps leadership groups, working teams and organizations to build sustainable capacities in collaborative learning and relationship-centered care. Williamson is currently involved in several long-term projects including, a Relationship Centered Care Initiative at Indiana University School of Medicine, a staff-development initiative at the American Board of Internal Medicine, and leads *The Courage to Lead*, a personal and professional development program for health care leaders.

INDEX

AAMC (Association of American Medical Colleges), 6, 12, 25, 88, 90, 96, 104, 111, 136, 214, 233, 235, 240

ABIM (American Board of Internal Medicine), 6, 12, 25, 30, 90, 104, 135, 136, 188, 189, 233, 234, 235, 240

ACGME (Accreditation Council of Graduate Medical Education), 6, 12, 13, 43, 45, 46-47, 48-55, 57, 90, 104, 157, 178, 189, 190, 197, 208, 216, 217, 228, 233, 235, 240, 241

ACP (American College of Physicians), 46, 104, 167

Administrators, 12, 19, 68, 107, 139, 140, 145, 195, 200, 244

Altruism, 9, 10, 13, 15, 16, 17, 25, 27, 29, 34, 38, 65, 70, 103, 105, 108, 110, 112, 124, 129, 134, 136, 170, 172, 175, 188, 219, 220, 235, 236, 237

AMA (American Medical Association), 12, 35, 46, 117, 118, 173

Autonomy; patient, 15, 34, 131; professional, 10, 12, 13, 15, 16, 31, 32, 33, 34, 35, 133, 141, 206, 219

Behavior(s), 5, 6, 19, 27, 28, 29, 37, 45-46, 63, 64, 67, 72, 88, 90, 94, 97, 98, 103, 105, 106, 107, 110-113, 116, 119-123, 124, 131, 135, 138, 140, 159, 167, 170, 171, 172, 173, 175, 180, 182, 186, 187, 190-193, 194-196, 201, 213, 216, 224, 226, 228, 230, 233, 234, 235-238, 239-241, 242-246, 247

Boundaries, 17, 52, 73, 130, 133, 141, 146, 225, 257

Care, 13, 15, 17, 35, 38, 39, 44, 50, 51, 52, 66, 67, 72-76, 78, 79, 112, 115, 117, 122, 144, 145, 153, 172, 181, 182, 186, 187, 188, 189, 197, 214, 216, 217, 218, 220, 221, 224, 228, 229, 237, 239, 246, 257; end of life, 189, 200, 206; ethics of, 130

Casuistry, 141, 142, 143

Commercialism, 9, 11, 12, 14, 16-19, 78, 79, 166, 213

Collaboration/Communication, 43, 46, 55, 56, 57, 71, 72, 73, 105, 106, 135, 141, 145, 167, 175, 176, 177, 182, 188, 189, 190, 197, 213, 216, 218, 224, 225, 229, 242, 256

Community, 26, 28, 29, 33, 35, 37, 38, 39, 40, 63-78, 83, 96, 113, 117-118133, 134, 138, 139, 143,